The Complete Guide to MRCPsych

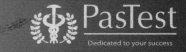

PasTest
Dedicated to your success

The Complete Guide to
MRCPsych

by

Nicholas Taylor

James Reed

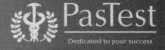
PasTest
Dedicated to your success

First Published 2006

ISBN: 1904 627 730
ISBN: 978 1904 627 739

A catalogue record for this book is available from the British Library.

The information contained within this book was obtained by the author from reliable sources. However, while every effort has been made to ensure its accuracy, no responsibility for loss, damage or injury occasioned to any person acting or refraining from action as a result of information contained herein can be accepted by the publishers or author.

PasTest Revision Books and Intensive Courses

PasTest has been established in the field of postgraduate medical education since 1972, providing revision books and intensive study courses for doctors preparing for their professional examinations.

Books and courses are available for the following specialties:

MRCGP, MRCP Parts 1 and 2, MRCPCH Parts 1 and 2, MRCPsych, MRCS, MRCOG Parts 1 and 2, DRCOG, DCH, FRCA, PLAB Parts 1 and 2, Dental Students, Dentists and Dental Nurses.

For further details contact:

PasTest, Freepost, Knutsford, Cheshire WA16 7BR

Tel: 01565 752000   Fax: 01565 650264

www.pastest.co.uk   enquires@pastest.co.uk

Text prepared by Carnegie Book Production, Lancaster

Printed and bound in the UK by MPG Books Ltd, Bodmin

To Thomas

Contents

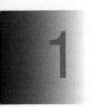

General revision techniques

This brief chapter aims to cover a range of important issues that you should bear in mind when planning your revision and actually revising.

By this stage in your career, you will have demonstrated a remarkable ability to pass exams. You have been successful at school and at medical school, and therefore must possess both raw ability and the knowledge of how to work effectively to meet deadlines and pass exams. Despite this, it is still useful to remind yourself of the basics of revision techniques, because it is likely to have been several years since you passed your last exam. It may be that your last exam was at medical school, where you were surrounded by people in a similar position and were revising without having to go to work on a daily basis, and perhaps look after a house and a family.

The most important thing to do in your revision is to make an early start and prepare yourself. Reading this book is an excellent way to do this!

You will hear many different opinions about how long it takes to revise for the MRCPsych Part I and Part II exams. Some people will claim that they revised only for a matter of weeks before passing. Others will have been revising for years, and still fail the exam time after time. There is no right or wrong length of time to allow for revision. It depends on your personal and family circumstances, as well as how busy your job is and how much time you have to revise at work, home and weekends.

As a rough guide, it is recommended that you start to think about your revision (for Parts I and II) about 6 months before each exam. The most important decision is actually to take the exam and take it seriously. You hear a lot of people saying 'I'll just have a go and see how I get on', and these people usually fail. Taking the exam is an expensive business, in financial terms, with fees of £500–600, and in terms of time and emotional commitment. If you are preparing properly, your revision may well have an effect on your social and family life, as well as your bank balance.

Start by familiarising yourself with the format of the exam and to collect revision materials. Find out who else is sitting the exam in 6 months' time and arrange to meet and talk about revision. Find the most popular websites and bookmark them in your browser. Set aside an area at home, and at work if you can, where you can gather your revision materials together. Have a look at the revision courses that are available and make sure that you book well ahead, to avoid last-minute disappointment. Revision is difficult enough without finding out that the revision course towards which you have been working is already full. Get hold of, and print off, the curriculum (available on the College website in the 'Training' section, under 'Examinations', then 'Regulations and curricula'). Make sure that you have the necessary books, both textbooks for general reading and, critically, books of past questions and answers. It will also be helpful at this stage to start reading journals (some of which are listed below) when you have a few spare minutes at work. You do not have to make notes or read the whole journal cover to cover – just try to develop the habit of reading the occasional article whenever you have the time.

Of the many books available, the following are particularly useful for Part I:

- *The Concise Oxford Textbook of Psychiatry* by Gelder or *The Shorter Oxford Textbook of Psychiatry* by Gelder (which is longer)
- *Symptoms in the Mind* by Sims
- *The A-Z of the MRCPsych* by Taylor
- *MRCPsych Part I Practice Papers: ISQs and EMIs* by Taylor
- *MRCPsych OSCEs for Part I* by Zoha.

For Part II, the following are also useful:

- *MRCPsych Part II Practice Papers: ISQs and EMIs* by Taylor
- *Companion to Psychiatric Studies* by Forrest, Freeman, Zealley and Johnstone
- *Critical Reviews in Psychiatry* by Brown and Wilkinson
- *Essential Revision Notes in Psychiatry for MRCPsych* by Fear
- *How to Read a Paper: The basics of evidence based medicine* by Greenhalgh
- *MRCPsych Patient Management Problems Explained* by Zoha
- *A Guide to Psychiatric Examination* by Aquilina
- *Critical Appraisal for Psychiatry* by Lawrie.

With regard to journals, the following are essential reading:

- *Advances in Psychiatric Treatment*
- *British Journal of Psychiatry*
- *Psychiatric Bulletin*
- *British Medical Journal.*

It is to be hoped that you will have access to these in your hospital library or online. Photocopy or print out any articles that seem particularly important or relevant and keep them in a lever-arch file, separated into topics by dividers. Many people find it helpful to outline the main points from each article in bullet points on sheets of paper in the file, for quick reference.

It is easy to spend a lot of time talking to colleagues, surfing the internet and buying books while convincing yourself that you are actually working. This is not the case and it is easy to slip into the work avoidance routine (or WAR) instead of actually getting down to it!

After all of this, there comes a point at which you must just start to do some work. Most people find it most productive to set a timetable for each week, and spend a set period of time each day working. How much time you can afford depends on your circumstances, but you should make a realistic and achievable timetable and stick to it, resisting the temptation to finish early on bad days, or even to work later on good days.

Make sure that you can revise somewhere quiet and (if possible) somewhere separate from your usual living or sleeping areas. If you can dedicate part of your home as a study during this time, this will be very helpful and allows you to leave all your work material in that one room. When you have finished your work, you can then take a break from work by leaving the room, and relax in an area that is completely 'work free'. There is nothing worse than spending a day revising before sitting down to relax and spotting a journal or book that you have not read on a table. Your anxiety levels will rise and your all-important relaxation will be interrupted.

The worst mistake that many people make is to work in or on their beds. This prevents you from switching off at the end of the day and 'contaminates' your bed (which should be a place of relaxation and calm) with thoughts of work and anxiety.

As the weeks go by, you should aim steadily to increase the amount of revision that you are doing each day, while still allowing time for relaxation at the end of the day. Make sure that you have regular breaks from your revision, and go for a brief walk (even if this is only around the table) during these breaks, to improve your concentration and get your blood flowing.

Some people find regular exercise, such as running, or a gym session, is an invaluable part of revision, and you should consider this, but avoid the temptation to spend your time exercising rather than revising.

Caffeine is another invaluable aid to many people. Used sensibly, it can increase concentration and ability to revise, but, used to excess, it can have exactly the opposite effect. Bear in mind the half-life of caffeine (look it up – it could be an ISQ!) and use it sensibly to avoid insomnia. Try to steer clear of energy drinks and caffeine tablets. If you're that tired, you probably need some sleep, or at least a rest, rather than trying to work when you're too tired to learn anything.

Alcohol also needs caution around exams. Many candidates do not drink alcohol at all, primarily for religious reasons, but, for those who do, it should be used carefully. Bear in mind the effect it has on sleep architecture, and the importance of sleep in laying down new memories. You need a reasonable quality as well as quantity of sleep if you are to feel refreshed and able to revise the next day. It may be best to use alcohol to relax in the evening, and to go to bed with very little residual alcohol in your system. Remember, 1 unit is cleared in 1 hour. If you go to bed with 4 units floating around, your critical deep sleep, which occurs early in the night, may be disrupted.

As the exam draws near, and anxiety levels rise, some candidates are tempted by a range of substances, including ß blockers, benzodiazepines and other drugs. Bear in mind that the effects of these prescribed drugs vary widely from one person to another, and you are better advised to find a non-pharmacological means of managing your anxiety. It is particularly dangerous to start using any sort of medication just before the exam because this can ruin your last few days of revision time if things do not go as planned, and these last few days can make all the difference between passing and failing.

Advice about revising for specific parts of the exam is given in the individual chapters, but some additional pointers may be useful here. Working in groups to cover as many individual statement questions (ISQs) and extended matching items (EMIs) as possible is invaluable. The same applies to practising the patient management problems (PMPs) in Part II – you should do this in groups as much as possible, 'revising' PMPs on your own is largely a waste of time. Practise as many PMPs as you can with specialist registrars and consultants in exam conditions before the exam because this will help you develop your technique and the exposure will reduce your anxiety. Long case practice is also valuable, with as many specialist registrars and consultants as you can find.

Revision courses vary widely in quality, duration and price, but all have something to offer. Talk to colleagues and find out which course will be most useful to you. It is important that you put in the work before going to the course because this will enable you to get the most out of it and will also boost your confidence.

Practice courses for the clinical exams are perhaps the most useful of all revision courses because they allow you to sit a complete mock exam under actual exam conditions and get feedback on your performance. The danger of these courses is that they often occur shortly before the real exam, and any negative feedback can lead to feelings of anger and despair.

In summary, plan your revision in advance, revise on your own and in groups, use as many sources of material as possible (with an emphasis on practice questions) and practise as much as possible in conditions as close to the real exam as possible. You will then make the most of your revision time. Good luck!

2 Individual statement questions and extended matching items (Parts I and II)

Format of the examination

Individual statement questions (ISQs) and extended matching items (EMIs) are found in Parts I and II of the exam.

In Part I, ISQs and EMIs form the whole of the written paper, and in Part II there are two ISQ/EMI papers: the Basic Sciences paper and the Clinical Topics paper.

ISQs, as their name suggests, are simply statements that are true or false. It is widely believed that the College has a very large bank of questions, from which it selects a variety for the exam each year. A limited number of questions are withdrawn for every new exam and replaced with new questions, but the majority remain the same over many years. This means that the same questions are asked repeatedly, which has important implications for revision. EMIs consist of a list of options, followed by a list of questions, clinical situations or descriptions, each of which has to be matched with the correct option from the initial list.

The College introduced EMIs relatively recently and they form an important part of the exam. They are given disproportionate weight in the marking, and each answer that you give to an EMI counts for 3 marks, compared with 1 mark for each ISQ.

There is no negative marking in the exam, so it is important to answer every question.

Revision techniques

Many candidates find that preparing for this part of the exam is relatively straightforward. The paper is a simple test of knowledge and revision is a simple learning of facts. One problem is that the range of subjects liable to be tested in the exam is very wide. It is important to get hold of the curriculum, which can be found on the internet by searching for a document called 'cr95.pdf' (originally published by the College as *Council Report*

95). The curriculum makes clear which subjects cannot be tested in Part I. A brief glance at it will make it clear that a high proportion of the material can be tested only in Part II.

In preparing for Part I, consider printing out the curriculum and crossing (or cutting) out all the subjects that can be tested only in Part II. You are left with a much more approachable list of topics and you must have some basic understanding of all the concepts covered.

ISQs and EMIs are a simple test of knowledge. It is tempting, therefore, to try to prepare for this examination by reading textbooks. In reality, this is a useful but limited part of the preparation that you will need to do. It is quite possible to read a large number of textbooks in great detail over many months and to fail the exam regardless. Knowledge of questions asked in previous years is invaluable because, quite often, the same questions will be asked on your exam day.

The first important rule for your revision is that you should spend a high proportion of your revision time looking at past questions and practice papers.

If you are revising in a hospital with a large number of other trainees, you will have access to their knowledge and expertise. There may be lists of past questions circulating and it is important to photocopy these and look up the answers. In many cases, previous candidates will have indicated their answers (true/false) on the sheet of paper. It is important not to accept these answers at face value because many of them are likely to be wrong. The last thing that you want to do is to learn incorrect answers to questions. By far the most productive way to revise is to attempt to answer the questions yourself and look up the answers to any questions that you do not know. In this way, you will revise your areas of weakness most thoroughly and quickly reinforce the areas with which you are familiar.

Although this is certainly the most efficient way to prepare for the ISQ/EMI papers, you may find that it is very time-consuming and disheartening when you start revising, because you will find yourself looking up the answers to the vast majority of questions. It can be off-putting to find that you have answered only a handful of questions after an hour of revision and you may feel that you are wasting your time. The truth is, of course, that revision is time-consuming, especially when you first start, as you will be unfamiliar with the material. After a few weeks or months of work, you will find yourself flying through the questions without needing to look up very much.

So, despite initial frustrations, persevere and be encouraged that you are in fact targeting your revision to those areas of your greatest weakness and learning an enormous amount of the most relevant material in the process. Nothing is more satisfying than sitting in the real exam and recognising many of the questions, remembering what you have read about them previously and answering them quickly, correctly and with confidence. Getting there is a long process.

Old photocopied papers with lists of questions are invaluable, but a more authoritative source of previous questions and answers can be found in one of the many books of ISQ/EMI questions and answers available commercially. It is important to use as many of these books as possible, particularly the more recently published works that are the most up to date. It may be possible to pass the EMI/ISQ part of the examination by learning past questions and answers from these books, although this approach is not recommended! This will not give you the depth of knowledge that is appropriate for the ISQ/EMI paper as well as for other areas of the exam and even your actual job as a psychiatrist.

If you are using some of the photocopied sheets of questions and answers that are passed around between candidates, be sure you don't place too much trust in the answers given on the sheet. These are often scribbled in the margin next to the question, and many of the answers are simply wrong. We would recommend looking up the answers to any questions that you are not absolutely sure about, because the very last thing you want to do is to learn the incorrect answers to questions that you will encounter in the real exam.

Make sure that you revise with the question papers and a large number of reference books available. You can then search for answers in the most appropriate book, which is readily to hand. Perhaps the most efficient way to find answers to obscure ISQs is by using the internet. By revising with a computer by your side and googling for particular words, you can find a definition or explanation more quickly than you could by looking through the index of a book. If you find computers slow or intimidating, or do not have a broadband connection, this may not be a possibility, but it really can speed up your revision.

The second important rule for maximising your revision productivity is that you should revise in groups if you possibly can. If you work in a hospital with a large number of other trainees, this will be easy, but, if you are relatively isolated, it is well worth travelling some distance to meet with others, at work or at home. Get together with three or four other candidates on a regular basis and take turns to ask and answer questions. You will revise more efficiently and for longer.

When revising in groups, you will usually find that at least one member of the group knows the answer to any given question and this is a very quick and efficient way to revise because you save on the time that you would otherwise spend looking up the answers to individual questions in textbooks. Alternatively, one member of the group can look up the answer in a textbook, or even on the internet, while the other members of the group carry on with their questions and answers. Revising in groups in this way is a good way to keep your motivation from failing when you are revising late at night or at the weekend. You often find that you are able to participate as a member of a group and stay motivated, when you would give up and go to bed if you were revising alone. As part of the general discussion, you will often hear little snippets of information that form the answers to other questions, which can be very valuable.

When revising, it is important to get hold of as many sample EMI questions as possible. The format for EMI questions is unlike anything that you will have seen before and can be quite counter-intuitive at first. Take time to answer as many EMIs as possible to get a feel for the range of subjects covered. Unlike the ISQs, EMIs are not reused in the exams, so you cannot hope to find exactly the same EMI in the real exam. What you will find is a selection of EMIs covering the same subjects.

When the exam is drawing near, it is very important that you take time to practise full mock exam papers, in exam conditions, sticking to the strict time limits of the real exam. You will need sensibly written, recent, practice papers to do this properly; ISQs and EMIs for both the MRCPsych Part I and the MRCPsych Part II are recommended. These books have questions, answers, explanations and references, all in the actual exam format, with several full practice papers, for both Parts I and II.

Examination technique

You will have discovered during your revision that time can be very short in the exam. In Part I there are 133 ISQs and 10 EMIs with an average of 3 questions in each. You have 90 minutes for the exam, which is an average of about 30 seconds per question.

It is recommended that you start by working your way right through the question paper from beginning to end, answering all the questions that you can answer immediately. Hopefully, this will be most of them! Put a faint pencil mark in the margin next to any questions that you cannot answer straight away, so that you can come back to them later.

There will be some questions that seem ambiguous, badly written or very difficult to understand. It is vital that you do not waste any time thinking about these questions. If you can't answer them after 20 seconds, put a mark in the margin and move on. There will be easier questions later in the paper on which you should spend time instead.

Once you have been all the way through the paper, go back to the start to check your answers and have another look at the difficult questions. Again, there is relatively little time, so, if you are still struggling with a question at this stage, it may be best just to make an intelligent guess and move on.

The papers are marked by computer; the College uses the computer to identify the top few per cent of candidates. These candidates' answers are analysed and any questions that they disagree on are automatically removed from the final marking. What this means is that the puzzling, ambiguous, difficult questions, which you could spend 10 minutes trying to answer (and still get wrong!), are likely not to be counted in the final marks in any case.

You are allowed 90 minutes for each ISQ/EMI paper and it is absolutely vital that you answer all the questions. Very few candidates who miss out questions manage to pass the exam.

The questions are given in a booklet and there is a separate answer sheet. You must make a mark with a pencil in the small boxes ('lozenges') on the answer sheet. All the answer sheets are fed into a computer, which marks them automatically. For this reason, your pencil marks need to be clear and preferably with an HB pencil. You must take a good eraser into the exam with you. If you do notice a mistake and want to change your answer, the original pencil mark needs to be erased thoroughly to avoid confusion. Consider buying an 'india rubber' from an art supply shop, because these erase pencil marks more easily than standard erasers and will do less damage to the paper.

Make absolutely certain that you have not missed a page in the question book, that you have made clear marks in the 'lozenges' on the answer sheet and that you have put a mark for every answer.

Note: The 'A–Z' referred to in the practice questions which follow is the PasTest publication *The A–Z of the MRCPsych* by Dr Nicholas Taylor.

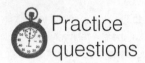

Practice questions

Sample ISQs

Part I

1 Echopraxia is a normal voluntary movement

1 F – it is an abnormal voluntary movement (A–Z, p. 129)

2 Depersonalisation/derealisation syndrome is associated with sensory deprivation

2 T – sensory deprivation can cause this syndrome (A–Z, p. 102)

3 Delirium tremens is characterised by haptic hallucinations

3 F – lilliputian hallucinations. Haptic hallucinations are superficial tactile hallucinations (A–Z, p. 95)

4 Ataxia is always caused by disease of the central nervous system

4 F – it can be caused by drugs such as benzodiazepines and lithium. Beware questions featuring the words 'always' and 'never'. The answer is (almost) always 'false' (A–Z, p. 45)

5 Perseveration is pathognomic of organic disorder

5 T – this is the only clinical feature in psychiatry that is pathognomic of anything, at least for the purposes of the MRCPsych exam (A–Z pp. 245–246)

6 Schneider was an object relations theorist

6 F – object relations theorists included Balint, Winnicott and Fairbairn. There were two Schneiders: Kurt, who described the first-rank (schneiderian) symptoms of schizophrenia, and Carl, who described a number of disorders of thought including fusion, drivelling and omission. Several questions will invite you to confuse Carl and Kurt Schneider.

7 Secondary delusions can be explained by other symptoms

7 T – they occur as a result of other problems such as delusional mood (which is also known as *wahnstimmung*)

8   Dementia causes patchy cognitive impairment
8   F – the loss is global.

9   Intact memory requires two of the following: encoding, storage and retrieval
9   F – it requires all three (A–Z p. 205)

10   Tranylcypromine is a hydrazine compound
10   F – it is a non-hydrazine monoamine oxidase inhibitor

There are lots of questions about drugs and which class of drugs they belong to. This information is in all the textbooks as well as the BNF (*British National Formulary*) and needs to be learnt, for easy marks. There will be at least a couple of this sort of question in every Part I and Part II exam.

Part II – Clinical Topics

1   Depressive episodes can be precipitated by phenothiazine antipsychotics

1   T – antipsychotics most often act to elevate mood, but phenothiazines can have the opposite effect, along with many other drugs (A–Z, p. 103)

2   Gradual onset of symptoms in schizophrenia indicates a better long-term prognosis

2   F – sudden onset is associated with a better prognosis

There are many questions looking at factors affecting the prognosis in schizophrenia and risk factors for suicide in schizophrenia.

3   The lifetime risk of schizophrenia is higher when both parents have it, compared with having one affected parent and one affected sibling

3   T – the risk is 46% as opposed to 17%

4   Bulimia nervosa includes a morbid fear of fatness, with the weight threshold set below the ideal weight

4   T – in this sense, it is similar to anorexia nervosa

The clinical features of anorexia and bulimia nervosa are particular favourites of examiners, and there are long lists of these that need to be learnt.

5   Organic psychosis can result from hypothyroidism

5   T – this is the most common psychiatric disorder resulting from hypothyroidism

6   Borderline personality disorder is often associated with saddened affect

6   T – at least intermittently

7   Depersonalisation can be pleasant

7   F – it is unpleasant by definition

8   General paralysis of the insane occurs within 3 years of initial infection

8   F – it occurs at least 5 years after infection with syphilis

9   Brain fag syndrome is seen most commonly in southern Europe

9   F – it is seen in Africa and results from excessive anxiety at the time of exams

10   Hyperparathyroidism can cause renal colic

10   T – caused by electrolyte imbalance

Part II – Basic Sciences

1 Barbiturates and methadone are class B substances

1 F – methadone is a class A substance; barbiturates are class B

2 The spino-olivary tract conveys information relating to joint position

2 T – proprioception and cutaneous sensation

3 The various leadership styles are equally effective, regardless of the task that needs to be completed

3 F – some styles, such as autocratic leadership, are better suited to crisis situations

4 Double-blind studies were first described by Bateman

4 F – Bateson described double-blind communication, which occurs when conflicting messages are communicated at the same time by different methods, such as telling a child that he or she has done well while looking irritated. Double-blind studies involve neither the researcher nor the subject knowing what intervention the subject has been given. Several exam questions aim to confuse the two

5 Baumeister described belongingness as a fundamental need

5 T – Baumeister and Levy (A–Z, p. 57)

6 Beck's cognitive triad involves a negative view of oneself, others and the universe

6 F – oneself, current experience and the future

7 Grandiosity is a psychotic defence mechanism

7 T – there are many questions about defence mechanisms, including their classification into primitive and sophisticated, as well as questions about who originally described them and which were classified as 'psychotic' by Klein

8 About 50% of the cerebral cortex is composed of neocortex

8 F – about 90%

9 Antipsychotic-induced pyrexia is usually dose related

9 T

10 Signal detection theory states that perception is based entirely on stimulus intensity

10 F – it states the opposite: that the biological and psychological contexts of the perception are important

Sample EMIs

1   Theme: EEG phenomena

A   δ Rhythms

B   Waves

C   γ-Hydroxylase

D   Flat trace

E   λ Rhythms

F   α Rhythms

G   κ Rhythms

H   Spikes

I   μ Rhythms

J   β Rhythms

Choose the EEG phenomenon from the list above that is most closely associated with each of the following statements:

1   The characteristic frequency is 8–13 Hz

2   This is the fastest feature commonly seen on the normal EEG

3   Occurrence of this feature relates to eye movements during visual inattention

Answers:
_____

1   F – α rhythms

2   J – β rhythms (with a frequency of between 13 and 30 Hz)

3   E – λ rhythms (which are occipital in origin and occur only when the eyes are open)

2   Theme: eriksonian stages

A   Integrity vs Despair

B   Intimacy vs Isolation

C   Initiative vs Guilt

D   Sensorimotor vs Preoperational

E   Identity vs Confusion

F   Industry vs Inferiority

G   Generativity vs Stagnation

H   Trust vs Mistrust

I   Phallic vs Oedipal

J   Autonomy vs Shame and Doubt

Identify the stage from the list above described by Erikson as involving the following:

1   Seeking of independence from parents, leading to improved self-esteem

2   Occurrence between the ages of 40 and 64 years

3   Failure at this stage leads to suspicion, insecurity and fear in the future

---

Answers:

1   J – Autonomy vs Shame and Doubt

2   G – Generativity vs Stagnation (when attempts are made to continue growth and contribute positively to society)

3   H – Trust vs Mistrust (success in this stage leads to trust in the external environment and a sense of hope)

3   **Theme: lobes**

A   Pseudoagnosia

B   Reduced appreciation of music

C   Confabulation

D   Topographical agnosia

E   Klüver–Bucy syndrome

F   Mild euphoria

G   Gerstmann's syndrome

H   Reduced social awareness

I   Contralateral spastic paresis

J   Ipsilateral optic atrophy

From the list above, identify the function most closely identified with lesions involving the following areas:

1   Bilateral temporal lobe

2   Occipital lobe

3   Dominant parietal lobe

Answers:
_____

1   C – confabulation

2   A – pseudoagnosia

3   G – Gerstmann's syndrome (agraphia, dyscalculia, finger agnosia, right–left disorientation)

4   Theme: equivalence in developmental stage theories

A   Piaget's formal operational stage

B   Freud's oral stage

C   Erikson's stage of Integrity vs Despair

D   Freud's genital stage

E   Erikson's stage of Initiative vs Guilt

F   Erikson's stage of Generativity vs Stagnation

G   Freud's anal expulsive stage

H   Erikson's stage of Intimacy vs Isolation

I   Erikson's stage of Industry vs Inferiority

J   Freud's anal retentive stage

Choose the stage theory from the list above that is most associated with the same level of development as the following:

1   Erikson's stage of Trust vs Mistrust

2   Freud's stage of latency

3   Piaget's preoperational stage

Answers:

1   B – Freud's oral stage

2   I – Erikson's stage of Industry vs Inferiority

3   E – Erikson's stage of Initiative vs Guilt

5   Theme: hallucinations and illusions

A   Reflex hallucinations

B   Haptic hallucinations

C   Ecmnesic hallucinations

D   Third-person hallucinations

E   Hypnagogic hallucinations

F   Extracampine hallucinations

G   Running commentary

H   Lilliputian hallucinations

I   Visceral hallucinations

J   Functional hallucinations

Choose the most appropriate term from the list above for each of the following:

1   The hearing of high-pitched voices when a tap is running

2   Seeing very small people who do not really exist

3   The sensation that insects are crawling across the skin

Answers:
_____

1   J – functional hallucinations

2   H – lilliputian hallucinations (occur in delirium tremens)

3   B – haptic hallucinations

6   Theme: receptor antagonists

A   GABA-B (γ-aminobutyric acid B)

B   Acetylcholine receptors

C D_4-Receptors

D $5HT_1$-receptors

E   α-Adrenoceptors

F D_2-Receptors

G   GABA-A

H $5HT_3$-receptors

I   α-Receptors

J $β_1$-Adrenoceptors

Identify the specific receptor from the list above that represents the site of antagonism of each of the following substances:

1   Atropine

2   Flumazenil

3   Atenolol

Answers:

1   B – acetylcholine receptors (muscarinic)

2   G – GABA-A

3   J – $β_1$-adrenoceptors

7 **Theme: classification of psychotropic drugs**

A Clozapine

B Trifluoperazine

C Chlorpromazine

D Zopiclone

E Haloperidol

F Zuclopenthixol

G Amisulpiride

H Quetiapine

I Mianserin

J Risperidone

Choose the drug from the list above that belongs to each of the following classes:

1 Cyclopyrrolone

2 Aliphatic phenothiazine

3 Benzisoxazole

Answers:

1 D – zopiclone

2 C – chlorpromazine

3 J – risperidone

8 Theme: clinical features of grief reactions

A Sadness

B Sense of dejection

C Low socioeconomic group

D Feelings of self-reproach

E Stage 3 of a normal grief reaction

F Anger

G Unexpected grief syndrome

H Lindeman's morbid grief reaction

I Stage 2 of a normal grief reaction

J Numbness

Choose the term from the list above that is most closely associated with the following:

1 The type of grief described by Parkes as involving feelings of self-reproach and a persistent sense of the presence of the deceased

2 Resolution of symptoms, resumption of social activity and positive memories of enjoyable times

3 Stage 1 of a normal grief reaction

Answers:

1 G – unexpected grief syndrome

2 E – stage 3 of a normal grief reaction

3 J – numbness

9   Theme: conditioning

A   Operant conditioning

B   Unconditioned stimulus

C   Classical conditioning

D   Escape conditioning

E   Avoidance conditioning

F   Negative reinforcement

G   Higher-order conditioning

H   Conditioned response

I   Trial and error learning

J   Conditioned discrimination

Select the item from the list above that is most closely described by each of the following:

1   Also known as 'respondent learning'

2   Salivation in response to a bell in Pavlov's dogs

3   The development of a conditioned stimulus from a neutral stimulus that is paired with an established conditioned stimulus

Answers:

1   C – classical conditioning

2   H – conditioned response

3   G – higher-order conditioning

10 **Theme: idiographic personality theories**

A   Rogers' self theory

B   Kelly's personal construct theory

C   Attitude-discrepant behaviour

D   Incongruence

E   The Q-sort technique

F   The repertory grid technique

G   Freud's developmental stage theory

H   WAIS-III

I   Allport's trait approach

J   Freud's topographical theory of mind

Identify the item from the list above that:

1   Identified cardinal, central and secondary dispositions as personality traits

2   Represents the difference between the ideal self and the perceived self

3   Is used to assess changes in an individual's perception of self

Answers:

1   I – Allport's trait approach

2   D – incongruence

3   E – the Q-sort technique

3 Part I: the OSCE

What is an OSCE?

The Objective Structured Clinical Examination (OSCE) is a format of clinical examination that is becoming increasingly popular in undergraduate and postgraduate settings. The concept of an 'objective structured examination' was first described in those terms by Harden in 1975 for use in undergraduate examinations, and in many respects has changed little in its implementation from that originally described. They are now used to examine very many different subjects at undergraduate level, from traditional clinical subjects (eg medicine and surgery) through to more theoretical ones (eg therapeutics). The various Royal Colleges are beginning to follow suit, with OSCE-style cases replacing the traditional short and long cases in the MRCP and MRCS exams. The Royal College of Psychiatrists has to come to the OSCE relatively late, with the first exam of this type being run in 2003.

An OSCE consists of a number of individual tasks (or 'stations'), each of which must be completed in a set period of time. The stations are marked according to strictly defined criteria, which should be independent of the individual examiner and arranged in a specific structure. The strictness of these criteria does vary across different implementations of the OSCE, from very specific tasks in a checklist (eg 'the candidate greets the patient', 'the candidate asks the patient if he hears voices') to more general statements of ability (eg 'the candidate demonstrates ability at eliciting suicidal ideas').

The principal advantages of the OSCE are that the content of the stations can be standardised and controlled, and that the marking scheme can be specifically targeted at the areas deemed to be of most importance. This eliminates the perceived problems with a traditional clinical exam that success or failure can depend on the attitude or suitability of the individual patient or examiner rather than on the candidate's clinical skills. Every candidate will face a large number of different examiners and scenarios, so the influence of an individual station on overall performance is minimised.

The disadvantages are that OSCEs are an artificial situation, and some feel that passing such an exam is as much concerned with technique as with knowledge and skill. Given that all the encounters are with simulated patients (and therefore people who are mentally well), the experience of interviewing them cannot be entirely the same as with an individual who is genuinely unwell. In addition, the task-oriented nature and limited time can interfere with components of a normal interview such as building a rapport with the patient.

The Royal College view

The Royal College has published some limited guidance with regard to the OSCE. This begins by stating:

> The aim of the OSCE is to test your clinical and communication skills. It is designed so that an examiner can observe you putting these skills into practice.

The Part I OSCE consists of 12 stations, each lasting 7 minutes. Before each station, there is 1 minute for moving to the station and reading the instructions. The instructions are posted outside the station, but they are also available inside for reference during the exam. A bell will ring to indicate the beginning and end of the station, and also there is a bell at 6 minutes to give you a warning that time is almost up.

The College cites five main skills that the OSCE sets out to test:

1. History taking

2. Examination skills

3. Practical skills/use of equipment

4. Emergency management

5. Communication skills.

All the scenarios to be faced in the exam will fall into one of these categories, although clearly they are very broad, and can be imagined to cover most tasks carried out by an SHO (senior house officer) in psychiatry. The level of performance expected is that of a trainee who has completed 1 year of basic training, in both general adult and old age psychiatry. The knowledge base required for the written paper is also assumed, and some of the tasks may rely more heavily on that than on your clinical experience (such as explaining the principles of psychological treatments).

The marking scheme for the exam is important to bear in mind when approaching the exam. The checklist format described above is not used in the Part I OSCE (Oyebode, 2002). Instead, a list of objectives that the candidate should achieve is given on the mark sheet, and the examiner's task is to mark the candidate on each of these objectives using a 5-point scale (excellent, good, acceptable, borderline fail, very poor). The marks given are then subject to weighting, of which the examiner is unaware, for example, in a station concerned with history taking in depression the assessment of suicidal risk may be weighted highly. Hence, a poor performance on that particular task is likely to cause the candidate to fail, even if he or she has done well on the other objectives. This is in some ways advantageous, because a good performance on the key aspects of the station will lead to a good overall mark.

Preparing for the OSCE and revision technique

As with any exam, good preparation is the key to success. It is a mistake to assume (as some do) that there is no need to revise for a clinical exam. There are three main areas that require preparation: factual knowledge, psychiatric clinical skills and practical skills.

Factual knowledge

Despite being a clinical exam, you are required to have a good grasp of the facts that underlie clinical practice. Many of the stations involve explaining aspects of diagnosis and treatment to patients, and to do this well you clearly need to have a good understanding of the subject yourself.

It is a good idea to develop a structure for approaching a discussion of diagnosis or treatment, and use this structure to learn appropriate facts. The exact details of the structure are a matter of personal choice, and often in the course of clinical work you may have developed your own approach. An example of a framework for thinking about a diagnosis would be as follows:

- Exact name of illness

- Epidemiology (prevalence figures)

- Aetiology (common causes, heritability, role of substances)

- Common symptoms

- Options for treatment and their efficacy

- Prognosis (likelihood of future episodes, risk of relapse).

In developing your structure, remember that, in the exam itself, most of the discussion will need to be in lay language and so readily understandable. Your task is to communicate information to the patient or relative, not to impress the examiner with your detailed knowledge of the subject. It is therefore important to avoid using jargon, and always to be ready to give clear explanations of any medical terms used.

The role of substances (especially cannabis) in the aetiology of schizophrenia is a subject that has come up several times in the exam, so for all diagnoses it is important to consider what the impact of substances is likely to be. Remember to include alcohol, particularly when thinking about depression. When it comes to the exam, it is important to handle these subjects sensitively and in such a way as not to appear to be blaming the patient. This can be done with open questions such as 'How do you think alcohol affects you?' or 'Have you been drinking any more than usual lately?', rather than asking baldly (as candidates have been known to do) 'Do you drink too much?'.

Using a framework like this will provide a structure for thinking about the diagnosis and also for approaching discussion within an OSCE station. Remember that any discussion must be a two-way process, and not a 7-minute lecture! You should aim to prepare something along these lines for all the diagnoses that you are likely to encounter in day-to-day practice. The following would be a bare minimum:

- Depression (including postnatal)
- Bipolar affective disorder
- Schizophrenia and psychotic disorders (eg puerperal and drug-induced psychosis)
- Agoraphobia
- Generalised anxiety disorder
- Panic disorder
- Post-traumatic stress disorder
- Body dysmorphic disorder
- Anorexia nervosa
- Bulimia nervosa
- Dementia (Alzheimer's disease and vascular)
- Alcohol and drug dependence.

Similarly, for discussing treatments a similar framework can be used, such as the following:

- Name of treatment
- Type of treatment (drug, psychological therapy, biological therapy, etc.)
- How treatment is thought to work (effects on the brain, teaching coping strategies, etc.)
- How treatment is given (injection, tablet, 1:1 session with therapist etc)
- Procedure before starting (physical investigations, psychotherapy assessment, etc.)
- Indications for treatment (conditions for which the treatment is effective)
- Potential benefits (relief of symptoms, relapse prevention etc)
- Common side effects (those likely to be experienced etc)
- Rare but important side effects (life threatening, teratogenic etc)
- Potential risks associated (if not covered above, eg dependency).

Again, you will need to prepare something of this kind for all of the treatments that you might be asked about. You may not have directly encountered some of these (in particular the psychological therapies) in your training so far and this will need extra work. Again, in the exam you will need to discuss these in clear language and with the minimum of jargon. When explaining how treatments work, this must done in as simple a manner as possible and you should avoid using scientific terms such as 'neurotransmitter', 'receptor'.

In terms of which therapies to cover, the absolute minimum would be the following but you will probably want to add more as you go through:

- Drug treatments:
  - antidepressants (tricyclic antidepressants or TCAs, selective serotonin reuptake inhibitors or SSRIs, venlafaxine, etc.)
  - antipsychotics (typicals and atypicals, depots)
  - mood stabilisers (lithium, sodium valproate, carbamazepine)
  - anxiolytics (benzodiazepines, buspirone)
  - hypnotics (zopiclone, etc.)

- anti-dementia drugs (donepezil, memantine etc)

- antimuscarinic drugs used for relief of extra-pyrimidal side effects (procyclidine, etc.).

- Other biological treatments:

  - ECT (electroconvulsive treatment).

- Psychological treatments:

  - cognitive–behavioural therapy

  - interpersonal therapy

  - psychodynamic psychotherapy

  - exposure and response prevention

  - graded exposure

  - systematic desensitisation.

Remember that the task posed may involve any aspect of the treatment. There have been many stations that consist of simply explaining a particular treatment, but there have equally been many that approach the subject from a different angle. For example, one station was concerned with explaining the likely side effects of long-term venlafaxine and the patient was particularly concerned about possible sexual problems. Other stations have involved explaining to relatives the aspects of treatment (such as anti-dementia drugs), which requires a slightly different approach.

Psychiatric clinical skills

Given that OSCE stations are reasonably predictable and that the format of the stations is known, it is relatively straightforward to practice. Although you may be confident of your skills in your day-to-day work, the exam conditions of an OSCE are quite different and regular practice of working in those conditions will help enormously when you come to sit the exam.

As described above for tackling factual information, having a structure in your mind for approaching various clinical situations is very helpful. It is not possible to construct a 'standard' structure for approaching clinical problems as used above for diagnosis and treatment, but what you can do is look around for acceptable structured tools that are used in different situations. A simple example is the 'CAGE' questionnaire (Have you ever felt you should CUT down on your drinking; Have people ANNOYED you by criticising your drinking; Have you ever felt GUILTY about your drinking; Have you ever had an EYE opener (a drink on waking)?) used for assessing the possibility of an alcohol problem. The ICD-10 criteria for alcohol dependence provide a more detailed structure for approaching an alcohol history.

There are quite a number of topics (beyond straightforward history taking and mental state examination) that can be regarded as 'core skills', which are very likely to be tested. These would include:

- Assessment of suicide risk (Beck's Scale for Suicidal Intent, Pierce's Suicide Intent Scale)
- Assessment of capacity to consent (see Addendum III)
- Assessment of testamentary capacity (see Addendum III)
- Assessment of cognitive function (Folstein's Mini-Mental State Examination, Abbreviated Mental Test Score)
- Assessment of drug and alcohol dependence (CAGE questionnaire, ICD-10 criteria for alcohol dependence)
- Assessment of risk in cases of morbid jealousy.

For each of these there are a number of standard tools and approaches used for assessment (examples are given in parentheses). You will not be specifically tested on the use of these, but revising them beforehand and keeping them in mind should give you a basic structure for approaching these stations. Remember that, although standardised tools are helpful for providing a general structure, they should not be rigidly adhered to and you will need to respond to the patient as the station progresses. For a more general overview of the psychiatric interview, the 'Present state examination' gives a comprehensive list of questions for assessing every imaginable symptom. It is far too complex to learn in its entirety, but can be useful for developing an approach to the assessment of symptoms.

Morbid jealousy is a subject that has come up more than once and is deemed to be important because of the likelihood of risk to others – not only to the spouse, but also to the person with whom the patient feels that their spouse has been unfaithful. It is important to explore these aspects in detail.

Physical examination and practical skills

These are by far the easiest stations that you will meet – they are simple to prepare for and easy to practise. They are often much shorter than the others, many taking only a few minutes to complete. You should be prepared to examine any of the main systems of the body, although some (cardiovascular, nervous and locomotor) are of more relevance to psychiatry (in terms of drug side effects, etc.) and so more likely to be asked about. Other more specific skills are also tested including cardiopulmonary resuscitation (CPR), cranial nerve examination, funduscopy, assessment of extrapyramidal side effects and assessment of thyroid function.

The best source of information for approaching these stations are general medical textbooks. There are a number of books directed specifically at clinical examination (eg Epstein et al., 2003; Douglas et al., 2005), which are very helpful. You will not be asked to do any task that you will not already have covered at medical school, so it should largely be a case of revision rather than learning new skills.

Funduscopy is an area that many candidates worry about, although in fact it is one of the least common physical examination stations. The key to success in all these stations is to practise all the likely tasks in advance, so that on the day you can switch into a well-rehearsed routine. The most difficult aspect of these stations (in those using models or mannequins) is to remember to address the model as if he or she was a real patient, and talk him or her through the procedure. Some stations will ask you to present the findings to the examiner, so make sure that you remember to do so!

Putting it together

A distinct advantage of the OSCE from a candidate's point of view is that the predictable nature of the exam makes it easy to practise. Having done all the relevant individual preparation as described above, there is no substitute for practising OSCE scenarios with others. There are now many sources for sample OSCE questions and model answers, such as the PasTest book by Zoha et al., 2004, and also numerous websites (eg trickcyclists – see references). You may also wish to construct your own, as the process of doing so will give some insight into what the examiners will be looking for.

Many hospital trusts also provide OSCE courses as part of the local MRCPsych courses, and there are also revision courses provided by third parties. The experience gained from such practice is extremely useful. There is also a good chance that some of the scenarios that you meet in practice will come up in the exam itself.

On the day

No matter how much practice you have done or how confident you are in your skills, the prospect of sitting the real exam is bound to provoke anxiety. This is often made worse by hearing 'horror stories' of others' experiences, and also by not knowing exactly how the exam is going to be conducted.

At present, there are two cities where the OSCEs are held – London and Sheffield. A number of different venues have been used within these centres, and they are usually hospitals (such as Guy's Hospital in London) or conference venues. The usual rules of exams apply – you should book accommodation as soon as you find out where the exam is and arrive the night (or even better the day) before the exam. You will need to allow plenty of time for getting to the venue itself – if you miss the start you may not be allowed in. If possible, visit the venue the night before the exam to check the arrangements for parking, etc.

You will have been informed by the College, well in advance of the details of the venue, which cycle you will be taking and what time it starts. The whole day is divided into a morning and afternoon session, and within each session there may be at least two separate sittings that begin at different times. However, to prevent information about the stations leaking out, all the candidates for the session are required to arrive at the start of that session and wait for the time of their sitting. This means that you may have to wait at the venue for quite a long time for your exam to start. You are kept in a waiting room, and although refreshments are provided this can be quite a tense time.

No matter how objective any exam purports to be, making a good impression on the examiner will always improve your chances of a good mark. You should dress in a smart and professional manner, and treat everyone you meet with courtesy at all times. You will not be allowed to take much into the exam room, although you will be allowed to leave bags, coats, etc. at the door. You will be given a pad of paper and a pen which is collected from you when you leave.

When you enter each station, you will find the examiner and the simulated patient or relative. The role of examiner in most cases is to act purely as an observer and, unless specifically directed by the question, you should not address the examiner at all and should behave as if he or she is not there. When you first enter the station, you will be asked for your name and candidate number, but once you have given this information you should immediately address yourself to the patient and begin the task.

There are usually at least two separate 'cycles' (with different candidates) of OSCE stations that run independently of each other, and they are often in the same large room. The individual stations are held in small, temporary booths. These are grouped together, so that all the booths that you visit are close to each other and in one place. Looking around the hall you may see several of these groupings of booths, but you will stay within the same group for the whole exam. You will visit 12 of these booths.

The booths themselves have thin walls and are often rather cramped. There is often only just enough room for the examiner, actor and candidate, and the noise from the other stations may be clearly audible. The layout of the booths can also be confusing and it is not always clear which station to move to next. There are always several organising staff on hand to assist, but every exam brings with it stories of candidates missing stations or doing them in the wrong order. Although this may sound strange, it is very easy to make such mistakes when you are anxious.

Most of the stations involve a clinical interview with a simulated patient or relative (played by professional actors). There are a few physical examination stations when a practical task is set, and these may involve an actor or a model or dummy. An examiner is present at every station, but unless the instructions state otherwise he or she plays no active part except to ask for your candidate number at the beginning of the task. Sometimes you may be asked to describe your findings to the examiner, or present the results of an assessment.

Occasionally there will be rest or pilot stations in the circuit. Rest stations are simply gaps in which you will have no task to perform. Some find these a welcome break, whereas for others they are a frustrating delay. Pilot stations are for OSCE questions that are being tested, and do not count towards your final mark.

Dealing with actors

The actors are given a detailed briefing about the character whom they are to play, and there is sometimes guidance about when to reveal certain information. Depending on the task, they may have specific questions that they want to be answered. A common mistake is to consider that, because they are not 'real patients', the usual rules of clinical interviews do not apply. The resulting barrage of questions seldom goes down well and is unlikely to achieve a good result. The station should not at any point seem like an interrogation, and using quick-fire questions in an effort to extract as much information as possible virtually guarantees failure. Anecdotal evidence from those involved in preparing SHOs for the exam suggests that this is a major problem for some candidates.

Actors are trained to 'get into character' and as much as possible take on the persona of the patient. Often in feedback sessions they will refer to the character whom they were playing in the third person (eg 'John didn't feel that you listened to him'). If they take a dislike to your manner of interviewing, or do not feel that they trust you, they will not reveal all the information that they have. It is therefore important to take time to build a rapport with the patient, to demonstrate empathy, to use appropriate body language, etc. It may seem a tall order to do so and then work through the task in the space of a 7-minute station. However, if the simulated patient feels comfortable with you he or she will respond much better to your questions as the station progresses. The other aspect of this is that it demonstrates to the examiner your skills at dealing with patients. If you are able to put the patient at ease, treat him or her with respect and address his or her concerns and questions sensitively and competently then you will be well on your way to a good mark.

The pool of actors used is quite small, and if you have attended revision courses or practice OSCEs you may well see some familiar faces. They have a good understanding of what is required by the candidates, and are not easily tricked into revealing important information. A recent candidate reported asking one of the actors 'Is there anything else of importance that we haven't covered yet?', to which the actor retorted 'You're supposed to ask me questions to find that out!'.

Finally, it is important to remember that the actor's information is by no means comprehensive and often covers only the salient points of the task in question. You can to an extent gauge how important the question is by how well it is answered. More importantly, you can also judge which questions are not important because the actor may struggle to answer them. If you are getting nowhere with a line of questioning, it may be worth considering changing tack and exploring a different area.

Conduct of the station

General points

As the marking scheme is not a strict checklist, the examiner does have quite a degree of control over the way the marks are awarded. It is very important to make a good impression early in the station, because this will convince the examiner that you are a good candidate and they will award marks accordingly. Try to act in as calm and confident a manner as possible, however difficult this might be.

Everyone reacts to stress and anxiety in a slightly different way, and it is important to be aware of how you react so that you can compensate for it. Particularly important in an exam concerned with communication is your speech. Many people when anxious tend to speak rapidly (especially when there is information to be imparted), although for some the opposite is true, and their speech slows down dramatically. Similarly, volume of speech can also be affected – some tend to look down and mumble whereas others speak rather too loudly.

You should aim to speak clearly and steadily. This will not only make it easier for the patient to hear and understand you, but also allow you to think carefully about what you are saying as you say it. Remember also to maintain good eye contact with the patient so that you can respond to their cues. Reassuring responses from the patient (such as nods, etc.) will demonstrate that they are following you, and looks of puzzlement or confusion should alert you that something is wrong – although this does depend to a point on the nature of the task.

Reading the question

Before you go in to the station, you will have 1 minute in which to read the instructions, which are posted on the door outside the station. They vary widely in length and complexity, and may contain a detailed history or only a very brief vignette. The last few lines will always contain the details of the task to be carried out, and it is the execution of this task that will get you marks. Clearly, you will not gain marks for carrying out tasks not listed.

It is therefore a good idea to scan the last few lines before reading the whole scenario, so that you identify the important points as you read. You will be issued with a notebook and pen when you go into the exam, so you can make brief notes of the task and your initial impressions about how to approach it.

Reading the question and addressing the task in it is the most important aspect of passing any station. No matter how good your communication skills are, you will not pass unless you carry out the task requested.

Introductions

When you enter the station, you will see the examiner and the actor (or plastic model in some cases). You will need to tell the examiner your name and candidate number, but in most cases you will have no further contact with him or her. You should turn immediately to the patient and begin the task. It is always good practice to introduce yourself to the patient, as is taught from early days at medical school. To do this, you need to know not only whom the patient is but also whom you are.

The patient's name is usually given in the instructions, and you should make a note of this so that you can greet the patient by name. Some of the stations do not give the patient's name (as a result of an oversight by the College!), and in this situation you should simply ask them their name at the outset. It is also important to remember that you may not be dealing with the patient him- or herself but a friend or relative. If so, make sure that you know what the relationship is. If (for example) you start talking about the patient's daughter when it is actually his wife who is the patient, you are bound to upset him.

There appears to be a fashion at present for asking people by which name they wish to be called. Although the aim is laudable, such a question does take up time and may come as a surprise to the actor (after all, it is a not a question one would use in any other setting!). It is quite safe to address the person in the station as Mr or Mrs <name>, and many would consider this to be good practice in any case.

With regard to knowing whom you are, this may seem obvious but, given the short instructions, it can be difficult to be entirely sure what your role is and so how to introduce yourself.

Many of the usual signposts (such as the name of the consultant for whom you are working) are not available. In addition, most of the general public are not familiar with terms such as SHO. Reading lay accounts of interactions with doctors (such as the book by Diamond, 1999) shows that patients are often confused by jargon-laden introductions. An example of a safe choice would be to introduce yourself as:

'Dr <name>, one of the junior doctors working in psychiatry.'

This is simple, clear, easy to remember and can be used whatever the task.

Setting the scene

Having introduced yourself, it is equally important to describe what you are going to do and why. The temptation to launch into questions or a long speech immediately must be resisted, and instead you should briefly outline what you are planning to talk about (this will also demonstrate to the examiner what you have in mind). This should need no more than a few sentences, eg in a station concerned with explaining ECT, you might open by saying:

'The consultant has asked me to talk to you about ECT, so I was planning to explain what ECT is, what the potential benefits are and go through with you any questions you might have.'

This only takes a few moments, but clearly shows the structure that you are planning to use for the rest of the station.

Tackling the question

Once you have outlined the structure, you need to tackle the task itself. As described above, the OSCE is supposed to simulate a real clinical encounter and so you should behave as much as possible as you would in real life. Wherever possible you ask open questions and encourage the patient to talk as much as possible. Even if the station is concerned with imparting information, asking the patient what he or she already knows about the subject will give the patient a chance to highlight areas that he or she wishes to know about, and stops the station becoming a lecture rather than a conversation. This may also reveal much other useful information (such as hopes, anxieties, fears, misconceptions), and can be used to set the agenda for the rest of the conversation.

Exceptions to this rule include the physical examination stations that are focused largely on the actual task. It is important to try to engage patients and talk them through the procedure, but it is not usually necessary to spend time discussing symptoms, etc. In some particular stations (such as funduscopy) a plastic model is used. You are still expected to address the model as if it were a real person (complete with smile, attempts to build rapport, etc.), although this is not always easy as a result of the lack of response!

In other stations you may find it very difficult to engage with the patient (such as those involving patients with psychosis, angry relatives). Faced with this, some candidates resort to firing a barrage of questions for fear of not completing the task. However, doing this is not likely to win the trust or confidence of the individual. A professional and empathetic approach is much more likely to be successful. The exam is designed to test your ability to deal with such difficult situations. If you encountered this situation in clinical practice you would try to engage the patient and gain his or her trust before asking specific questions. Once again, trying to develop a rapport is critical – very often the relevant details will emerge by themselves as you build a rapport with the patient. Actors are specifically instructed to reveal certain information only if they feel comfortable with the candidate.

It is important to enter each station with an open mind about what the problems are, and be vigilant for cues from the patient that might lead you in a different direction to that which you had expected, eg one station concerned a risk assessment of a young woman in accident and emergency who had taken a small overdose. Although the station appeared to be simply concerned with suicide risk, the real point of the station was that she was the subject of severe domestic violence at the hands of a boyfriend who was misusing drugs. Her risk from this was much more important than suicide risk, and to concentrate on that alone would have missed the point (and most of the marks).

Finishing the station

As you go through the station, you should be constantly thinking about the time remaining. A warning bell sounds when there is 1 minute remaining. It is much better to finish the station off with some closing statements rather than stop suddenly mid-sentence when the time runs out. Again, although the exam is an artificial situation, you should try to behave as much as possible as you would in real life. In closing the interview, you should give the patient an opportunity to ask questions and check that he or she has understood what you have talked about.

It is just as important to make sure that you do not finish the task too early. Not only can this be rather embarrassing (with patient, examiner and candidate sitting in silence until the time runs out), but it also suggests that you may not have adequately addressed all the parts of the task. The physical examination stations can often take much less than the full time, but in all the others you should expect the task to last for most of the time available. If you do feel that you have completed the task, rather than ending early you could continue to talk to the patient about the issues raised in the station. You may even find that you have missed something important, which surfaces in the course of the conversation.

Multidisciplinary working is now universal in psychiatry, and in closing you may wish to talk about the possible involvements in other disciplines. You might make reference to the role of a community psychiatric nurse, occupational therapist or psychologist in their care. Take care to avoid abbreviations (such as CPN, OT, etc.) which the patient may not have encountered before.

Negotiating the exam

Once the initial shock of being in the exam has subsided (and if you have prepared adequately) you should be able to settle into the structure of the exam. After you have completed one station you will have an idea of what the rest will be like, so you should be able to keep calm and concentrate on the task in hand. Try not to think about your performance in previous stations or worry about what else might come up. Each station is marked independently of the others, so each new station allows you a fresh start. It is also easy to lose count of how many stations you have completed, and the announcement of the end of the exam may come as a (pleasant) surprise!

Conclusion

The Royal College OSCE is not an easy exam to pass, but it is one that can be thoroughly prepared for and practised. Unlike some aspects of the exam, the preparation is directly relevant to clinical practice and should help you to develop your clinical skills and knowledge. The key to succeeding in the OSCE is to have not only a thorough background knowledge but also the ability to respond well to unexpected situations – just as in real life!

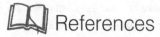 References

Diamond JC. *Because Cowards Get Cancer Too* ... London: Vermilion, 1999.

Douglas G, Nicol F, Robertson C (eds). *MacCleod's Clinical Examination*, 11th edn. Edinburgh: Churchill Livingstone, 2005.

Epstein O et al. *Clinical Examination*, 3rd edn. St Louis, MO: Mosby, 2003.

Harden RM, Stevenson M, Downie WW, Wilson GM. Assessment of clinical competence using objective structured examination. *BR Med J* 1975; i: 447–451.

Oyebode F. Commentary. *Advances in Psychiatric Treatment* 2002; 8: 348–350.

www.trickcyclists.co.uk

Zoha M, Kaligotla S, Wise J. *MRCPsych OSCEs for Part I*. Knutsford: Pastest, 2004.

Addendum I: common scenarios

As described in the text, the OSCE is a relatively predictable exam. There are certain topics that are very important, and that have featured in the exam on numerous occasions. Sometimes, even the wording of the question changes little from exam to exam!

Given below are a selection of popular OSCE stations, all of which have appeared in the exam in one form or another. This list is by no means exhaustive, but you should expect to encounter at least some of these in your exam. The descriptions given are deliberately brief, and should encourage you to think about how the scenario might be presented and what your approach could be. You may wish to use these as basis for your own revision.

History taking

- Taking a history from a patient with symptoms of anorexia nervosa
- Taking a history from a new mother (to include depressive and psychotic symptoms)
- Taking a history of alcohol use, particularly looking for symptoms of alcohol dependence syndrome
- Taking a history from the wife of a patient recently diagnosed with dementia to establish what the cause of the dementia is most likely to be
- Taking a history of a patient with PTSD (post-traumatic stress disorder), aiming to differentiate it from other anxiety disorders
- Taking a history of substance misuse and associated factors from a heroin addict.

Examination skills

- Assessment of capacity to consent
- Interviewing a patient suffering delusions, establishing the delusional nature of his or her ideas
- Interviewing a patient suffering hallucinations, establishing the exact nature of the hallucinations
- Assessment of cognitive function.

Practical skills/use of equipment

- Examine the locomotor system for extrapyramidal side effects
- Examine the thyroid of a patient taking lithium
- Examine the cranial nerves.

Emergency management

- Assessment of a patient in A&E after a suicide attempt
- Discussion of an assessment of such a patient with the consultant on the phone
- Discussion of management options with the relative of an elderly patient found wandering the streets

Communication skills

- Explain psychological therapies for the treatment of anxiety disorders
- Explanation of strategies for further drug treatment in treatment-resistant depression
- Explanation of options for management of bipolar affective disorder
- Explain ECT to a patient, and go through the process of obtaining consent
- Explanation of the diagnosis of schizophrenia to a relative of a newly diagnosed patient
- Explanation of anti-dementia drugs to a relative of a patient
- Discuss with a patient the possibility of taking long-term antidepressants, and the pros and cons of doing so.

Addendum II: common mistakes/pitfalls

- Failing to develop a rapport with the patient
- Speaking too quickly or too slowly
- Using medical jargon without adequate explanation
- Going into unnecessary detail
- Not carrying out the task detailed in the question
- Being rude to the patient
- Appearing to blame the patient (eg 'this happened because you are using too many drugs').

Addendum III: assessments of capacity

Capacity to consent

To have the capacity to give consent (eg for a medical procedure), the following conditions must be met:

1. The person must understand the information that has been given to him or her.

2. He or she must believe it to be true (this may not be the case in someone suffering delusions).

3. He or she must be able to retain the information (this may not be the case in someone with dementia or amnestic syndromes).

4. He or she must be able to weigh up the pros and cons of the options available and come to a decision.

It is important to note that in any situation the doctor who is giving a particular treatment is responsible for checking the patient's capacity.

Testamentary capacity

This term refers to the ability to make a valid will. The person making the will must be of 'sound mind' at the time of making it. This is judged according to four criteria:

1. Whether the person understands what a will is, and what the implications of making one are.

2. Whether the person understands the nature and extent of their property (ie what they own and its value). Detailed knowledge is not needed, but a general understanding is important (eg hundreds, thousands or millions of pounds).

3. Whether the person knows the names of his or her relatives, and can make a judgement about claims to the property.

4. Whether the person is free from any abnormality of mind that could influence the content of the will. The presence of an abnormality is significant only if it is likely to influence the will directly – simply having symptoms of mental illness does not automatically preclude an individual from making a will.

4 Part II: the critical review

What is a critical review?

Critical review or critical appraisal is one of the central pillars of the 'evidence-based medicine' movement. The term describes the skill of considering a piece of evidence (usually a research paper) in detail and assessing its strengths and weaknesses. The quality of the scientific method and design is considered, and also the relevance of the work to clinical practice. The purpose is not to identify every single fault in the evidence and use this as a basis for dismissing it; instead, a balanced approach should be taken in which strengths and weaknesses are assessed and a final conclusion reached.

The principles of evidence-based medicine are taught at all levels of training from medical school onwards. However, in spite of this there is a perception that many doctors do not exercise skills in this area and that clinical practice is often not based on the best available evidence. The purpose of the critical review paper in the MRCPsych exam is to raise awareness of the area, test some of the skills and, in particular, look at the application of research evidence to clinical practice. However, in order to pass the exam you do not need to have an in-depth knowledge of the process – instead, you will need a general understanding of the principles involved and an ability to extract information in response to specific questions.

The aim of this chapter is not to teach you the principles of critical review, but to describe the structure of the exam, outline strategies for approaching it and provide some revision of essential facts.

The Royal College view

The critical review paper was introduced in 1999, when it replaced the previous 'short answer' paper. The College has produced 'Guidance to candidates', which can be found in the recent College book *Critical Reviews in Psychiatry*. The guidance states that:

The Critical Review Paper is intended to assess skills and expertise which are not assessed in other parts of the MRCPsych Part II Examination ... Candidates will need to be aware of the science of research methodology and be skilled in the application of this.

Many candidates worry that they will be asked to produce a long and detailed appraisal of a paper. This is not the case; in fact, the exam consists of a relatively large number of focused and structured questions, many of which do not directly relate to the process of critical review. Many of the questions asked can be answered purely from factual knowledge, and the remainder depend on an ability to interpret data and graphs provided in the question.

Preparation for the critical review paper

As with all parts of the exam, a certain amount of background knowledge is required as well as some essential skills.

Knowledge

The knowledge required comprises basic facts about research methodology and some of the principles of evidence-based medicine.

Research studies can be of many different kinds and knowledge of the different types of study is essential. The most important of these are randomised controlled trials (RCTs), cohort studies and case–control studies, although others (such as qualitative research and economic analyses) have occasionally featured in the exam. As a minimum, it is important to know how each type of study works and the key strengths and weakness of each design. It is also important to understand the various types of bias to which each is susceptible. Bias (otherwise known as systematic error) can be defined as a difference between results obtained and the true situation, and also describes systematic processes that can lead to such a difference. These can be of many different types, eg publication bias refers to the fact that studies with positive findings are more likely to get published, so that a review of the literature may reveal a disproportionate number of positive findings.

Systematic reviews are a special type of study that methodically review all the published work on a particular subject. They often involve complex statistics that 'pool' all the available data to produce an overall indication of the effect (or lack of effect) of the subject being studied. You do not need to know the details of the statistical methods used, but you will need to be familiar with the way that the results are presented and be able to interpret them.

A basic understanding of statistical methods is required, and this is an area that provokes a great deal of anxiety. However, in-depth knowledge of statistical tests is not required and you will certainly not be expected to carry out any tests (such as t-tests, χ^2 tests) in the exam. You may, however, be asked to interpret the results of such tests, so it is important to be familiar with the way that they are presented. As a bare minimum, you should have an understanding of t-tests, analysis of variance (ANOVA), regression techniques, χ^2 tests and the Mann–Whitney U-test. It is beyond the scope of this book to give a detailed discussion of these techniques, which are covered in detail in other texts (see References).

Along with statistical methods used in research, there are a number of other calculated measures that are used as part of the process of critical review. These are usually simple figures that can be derived from data provided in research papers. These can be broadly divided into two groups:

- Those concerned with studies of diagnostic tests:

  - sensitivity

  - specificity

  - positive and negative predictive value

  - likelihood ratio

  - pre-test and post-test probability.

- Those concerned with studies of treatment:

  - absolute and relative risk reduction

  - number needed to treat

  - number needed to harm

  - odds ratio.

All these measures are relatively simple to calculate, and you will be expected to do so in the exam. The formulae are fairly easy to learn, and as a result these questions can provide quick and easy marks. A list of the relevant formulae is provided in Addendum I. The exam regulations advise taking a calculator into the exam, although it is important to check that your calculator does not breach regulations by having textual/graphic display, etc. If in doubt, basic calculators can be bought very cheaply from stationery shops.

Part of your preparation should involve reading around the subject. There are a number of books available that specifically target critical review in psychiatry, but more general books about evidence-based medicine are also very helpful. Greenhalgh's book *How to Read a Paper* is an excellent and readable introduction to the subject, and should be read by everyone preparing for the critical review paper.

Skills

The skills required for this paper are concerned with assessing the quality of the evidence presented and judging what (if any) relevance it has to clinical practice. A key part of this is looking out for errors in methodology and design, which will may call into question the conclusions made or invalidate them altogether.

The area of application of research to clinical practice is one that the College considers to be very important, and all of the critical review papers will contain questions on this. Allied with this is the ability to consider further research that might be helpful, either to confirm the results of the study or else to expand upon it.

Practice

Again, as with all exams one of the most important components of preparation is practice. As should be made clear by this chapter, technique and particularly timing is extremely important in this exam and this can be improved only by practise under exam conditions. Sample papers with answers are available from the College. The recent third edition of *Critical Reviews in Psychiatry* contains the past papers from 1999 to 2003, again with answers. Regular practice of these papers under exam conditions and against the clock will give you excellent experience, which will be very useful on the day. Only by this kind of practice will you gain a feel for the type of questions that are asked and become skilled at answering them.

In your day-to-day work you should have the opportunity to attend journal clubs and other evidence-based practice sessions. There are also a number of good courses concerning evidence-based medicine techniques in general, and also for preparation for the exam in particular. Although it may be tempting to try to learn the bare minimum necessary to pass the exam, it is wise to use these opportunities to learn skills in critical review that will be useful throughout your career. It is important to be able to appraise evidence for yourself, rather than relying solely on the judgement of others.

Approaching the critical review paper

Many candidates report that the most difficult aspect of the critical review paper is completing it in time. There are a lot of questions to be completed in a relatively short period of time. If there are a total of 30 individual questions to be answered (which is not uncommon), then only 3 minutes per question are available – and this does not allow any time for reading the paper!

It is important to remember that this exam is peer referenced, ie the marking is done with reference to the performance of all the candidates taking the exam. Questions that are universally poorly answered, or fail to discriminate well between good and bad candidates, are often excluded from the marking, and as a result the pass mark itself may be relatively low. Some candidates have reported passing the exam despite having missed out or only partially answering many of the questions – although this is not recommended!

The key to passing the exam is therefore to spend as much time scoring marks as you can. As described above, many of the questions do not require much if any knowledge of the paper itself and can be answered immediately. Therefore, it is a good idea to begin answering the questions as soon after the start of the exam as you can, and spend only a short period reviewing the paper before you start. Not all the information provided in the paper will be asked about, so it is a better use of time to read the relevant part of the paper selectively once a question has been asked about it. This approach is the complete opposite of that used for the essay paper (see Chapter 5), where it is important to invest time in considering the questions before beginning.

As with any exam, it is vital to read the question carefully and answer only what is being asked. This is particularly important in this paper because of the lack of time available. Do not be afraid to skip over questions if you are having difficulty with them. It is not uncommon for questions to be worded obscurely, making it difficult to be sure what is being asked. If you are finding a particular question difficult, it is likely that others are as well. The questions may at times appear difficult (eg Q: 'What is main disadvantage of a univariate analysis?'), but can often be answered by simply stating the obvious. (ie A: 'Only one variable at a time can be considered'). It is a common mistake to read too much into the question and spend time trying to think of a 'clever' answer, when a simple approach is all that is required. It is also worth quickly looking ahead at the next question, to make sure that your answer does not incorporate the answer to that as well.

It is also important to pay attention to the number of marks available for each question. It is not worth spending a long time over a question that is worth only 1 or 2 marks, when you might able to score more easily on a simpler question (such as the strengths and weaknesses of a particular study design) that carries more marks. The number of marks available will also give you a clue as to the extent of the answer required. The question may specifically ask for 'five strengths and five weaknesses' for 10 marks, but it may be worded more vaguely such as 'what are the implications of the results'. In the latter case, the number of marks available will suggest the number of points that you need to make. You will not gain any extra marks for providing more answers than are asked for, so it is important not to waste time providing a long and detailed answer to a question that is worth only 1 or 2 marks.

As with all other aspects of the exam, simply because the exam is about critical review does not mean that your other clinical and theoretical knowledge is redundant. Your clinical knowledge may well be of relevance, especially in the questions about clinical application of data, eg questions may be asked about important clinical variables to consider in a particular study, or possible confounding factors.

On the day – the critical review paper itself

The critical review paper is the first paper on exam day and lasts for 90 minutes. It consists of two main questions (A and B), each of which deals with different pieces of evidence. The exam is very structured. Each of the two main questions is broken down into smaller questions, which are again broken down into a number of parts worth a few marks each. There are seven questions in Question A (worth 10 marks each) and three in Question B (again worth 10 marks each), giving an overall mark out of 100.

Question A

The College has stated that Question A consists of questions about the findings of the paper, its design, methodology and importance in relation to clinical practice. The question begins with a clinical scenario, which gives a brief overview of a case and usually poses a clinical problem. A paper is then identified that could potentially help address the problem. Rather than being given the whole paper, extracts are provided for you to read. The extracts are usually from the 'Method' and 'Results' sections. There is usually at least one table or graph illustrating the results.

There are two broad types of question asked. The first are general questions concerning the research methodology and definitions of various terms. These questions can apply to any paper, and can usually be answered from factual knowledge and with little if any reference to the paper itself. These might include:

Give five strengths and five weakness of this type of study.

To answer this question requires only knowledge of which type of study has been used (ie case–control, cohort). Once this is known, the standard lists of strengths and weaknesses of the various study types can be used. Addendum II contains the most important of these for the main study designs.

What other types of study could have been used? List one strength and one weakness of each.

This requires the selection of sensible alternative types of study, accompanied by the standard strengths and weaknesses of each:

Define positive predictive value.

Define what is meant by validity, and describe three types of validity

Define the 95% confidence interval.

Definitions of all of these can be found in any statistics or critical review textbook. These need to be learned and earn easy marks. An in-depth knowledge of mathematics is not required.

The second type of question refers directly to the paper. These questions vary widely from paper to paper, although there are some questions that are commonly asked.

What hypotheses were the authors of this study testing?

This question requires extraction of information only about the hypothesis from the paper.

Give five strengths and five weakness of the design of this study.

This questions refers to specific aspects of the study in question that are strengths or weaknesses. Your answer will clearly depend greatly on the study in the question, but you should always consider the size of the sample (is it too small?), the measures used (are they well-recognised and validated instruments?) and means of follow-up (how are patients followed up, and how are losses dealt with?) as possible sources of good or bad design.

From the figures in the paper, calculate number needed to treat (NNT).

Calculations such as this do occur quite frequently, so it is wise to be prepared for them. As described above, you may be asked to calculate one of a limited number of different measures, each of which has a different formula. The best way to prepare for these questions is to revise thoroughly and practise the application of the formulae beforehand. Once you are confident with them, these questions become a relatively straightforward way of gaining marks.

There are invariably one or more questions that relate the findings of the paper to the clinical scenario outlined at the outset. It is important therefore to keep this in mind as you go through the question, and be aware of factors that may increase or decrease relevance, eg the population used in the study may be completely unrepresentative of that from which the patient in the scenario is drawn, or else there may be major flaws in the method (such as an inappropriate control group), which make the findings much less likely to be valid in practice.

Question B

Question B is much shorter than Question A. A different study is presented, although it is also much shorter (often being only a brief introduction and a single graph or table). There may be some connection between the subject of the papers in Questions A and B but this is not always the case. The College has said that the questions within Question B may be concerned with 'the practice of evidence-based medicine' although this is not further explained.

There is not usually a separate clinical scenario for Question B, and as the extracts are much shorter the questions usually depend more on interpretation of results than comments on methodology. The results may be presented as either tables or graphs. Similar to Question A, the clinical application of the data is often asked about, although this is usually in general terms rather than in relation to an individual patient.

One approach that is sometimes described is that of attempting Question B before Question A. This is said to get Question B 'out of the way' quickly and allow you to concentrate fully on Question A. This does pose difficulties with time management – you will naturally tend to answer questions more fully at the start of the exam, so you may complete Question B in detail and then not have enough time to attempt Question A adequately. Remember that Question A carries the majority of the marks, and it is more 'mark efficient' to spend time on Question A than Question B. Candidates report that it can be difficult to change focus from one paper to the next when changing questions. Some candidates have reported passing the exam having attempted only Question A – but this is not a strategy to be relied on.

Conclusion

The critical review paper requires a combination of knowledge and skill, but has the advantage of being probably the most relevant to clinical practice of all the written papers. As a result, you should already be familiar with some of the knowledge and skills required and those you gain through preparation for the exam will be useful throughout your career.

Many candidates dread this paper, thinking that 'it's all about maths', 'there is too much to revise', 'you need to pull the paper apart', etc. It is hoped that the foregoing will have provided reassurance that none of these is true. The exam does pose a number of challenges (not least of which is the lack of time available), but with thorough preparation you should do well in this paper.

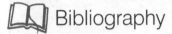 Bibliography

Brown T, Wilkinson G (eds). *Critical Reviews in Psychiatry*. College Seminars Series. London: Royal College of Psychiatrists, 2005.

This book is essential reading, because it contains the actual papers used from Spring 1999 to Spring 2004 with answers provided. There is also useful information about the exam itself.

Lawrie S, McIntosh A, Rao S. *Critical Appraisal for Psychiatry*. London: Churchill Livingstone, 2002.

This book is often recommended, but can be difficult to read and provides much greater detail than is required to succeed in the exam. It provides sample questions, but again these are very difficult. It is most useful if viewed as a reference book, rather than a tutorial.

Greenhalgh T. *How to Read a Paper: The basics of evidence-based medicine*. London: Blackwell Publishing, 2006.

This book is a very readable introduction to the principles of critical review. The discussion is pitched at a level that is easy to understand and very relevant to the exam paper. It also contains a very useful introduction to statistical terms.

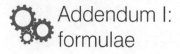 Addendum I:
formulae

Please note that the formulae below are for reference and explanations given are brief. Full discussion about the derivation and use of these formulae are beyond the scope of this book.

Diagnostic studies

Consider a study examining a diagnostic test for a disease. The test results are shown in the rows, with the columns showing the numbers of those with and without the disease.

	Disease positive	Disease negative	Total
Test positive	a	b	a + b
Test negative	c	d	c + d
Total	a + c	b + d	a + b + c + d

'a' is the number of those who tested positive and did have the disease (true positives).
'd' is the number of those who tested negative and did not have the disease (true negatives).
'b' is the number of those who tested positive and did NOT have the disease (false positives).
'c' is the number of those who tested negative and DID have the disease (false negatives).

$$\text{Prevalence} = (a + c)/(a + b + c + d)$$

Prevalence is the proportion of the whole population studied who have the disease. Thus,

$$\text{Sensitivity} = a/(a + c)$$

Sensitivity is the proportion of those people WITH the disease who are correctly identified by the test (ie test positive).

$$\text{Specificity} = d/(b + d)$$

Specificity is the proportion of those people WITHOUT the disease who are correctly identified by the test (ie test negative)

$$\text{Positive predictive value (PPV)} = a/(a + b)$$

Positive predictive value is the proportion of those people with a positive test who actually suffer from the disease.

Negative predictive value (NPV) = d/(c + d)

Negative predictive value is the proportion of those people with a negative test who do not actually suffer from the disease.

It is important to be aware that PPV and NPV are both affected by prevalence – as the prevalence decreases, the PPV drops and the NPV rises. This can make these measures unreliable in diseases with a very low or a very high prevalence.

Likelihood ratio of a positive result (LR+) = Sensitivity/(1 – Specificity)

With reference to the table:

LR+ = [a/(a + c)]/[d/(d + b)]

The likelihood ratio of a positive result is the probability that a particular result would be found in someone with the disorder than someone without. If the LR+ were 8, this would mean that the test result in question would be eight times more likely to be found in a person with the disease than in a person without the disease.

Likelihood ratio of a negative result (LR–) = (1 – Sensitivity)/Specificity

The likelihood ratio of a negative result is the probability that a particular result would be found in someone WITHOUT the disorder, rather than with it. Therefore, if the LR– were 5, this would mean that the result in question would be five times more likely to be found in a person without the disease than in a person with the disease.

Likelihood ratios can be used to calculate the post-test probability. This is similar to the PPV but is much less affected by the prevalence of disease. To calculate it mathematically, it is necessary to know the pre-test odds, which can in turn be calculated from the prevalence.

Pre-test odds = Prevalence/(1 – Prevalence) = (a + b + c + d)/1 – (a + b + c + d)

Post-test odds = Pre-test odds × LR+

Post-test probability = Post-test odds/(1 + Post-test odds)

Studies investigating treatment

Consider a study investigating the effects of a new drug versus placebo. The outcomes were expressed as improvement or no improvement.

	New Drug	Placebo	Total
Improvement	w	x	w + x
No improvement	y	z	y + z
Total	w + y	x + z	w + x + y + z

'w' is the number of those who took the new drug and did improve.
'z' is the number of those who took the placebo and did not improve.
'y' is the number of those who took the new drug and did not improve.
'x' is the number of those who took the placebo and did improve.

Experimental event rate (EER) = w/(w + y)

The EER is the proportion of those who took the new drug who improved (ie the 'event' is improvement and the 'experiment' is the new treatment).

Control event rate (CER) = x/(x+z)

The CER is the proportion of those who took the placebo (ie the control group) who improved.

Relative benefit increase (RBI) = (EER – CER)/CER

The RBI is the proportion by which the response is improved by taking the new drug. An RBI of 200% means that taking the new drug increases the response rate by 200%. If the study was looking at an intervention for reducing a risk rather than promoting a benefit, the result would be called the relative risk reduction (RRR).

Absolute benefit increase (ABI) = EER – CER

The ABI is the amount by which the new drug increases the response rate. Again, if the study were aimed at reducing risk the ABI is called the absolute risk reduction (ARR).

Number needed to treat (NNT) = 1/ABI

The NNT is the number of people who will need to be treated with the new drug in order to produce one extra response. It is always rounded up to the nearest whole number, because it is not meaningful to talk about fractions of a person, eg if the NNT was calculated as 7.2 it would be rounded up to 8. This would mean that eight people would have to be treated with the new drug for there to be one extra case of recovery, compared with placebo. Clearly, the ideal NNT would be 1 – every patient given the treatment shows improvement, although this is seldom seen in the psychiatric literature.

Odds ratio (OR) = $(w/y)/(x/z) = (w \times z)/ x \times x \times y)$

Odds are used as an alternative means of expressing the relationship between events. The odds of a particular outcome are the number of events (eg improvement) divided by the number of non-events (eg no improvement). In this case, the odds of improvement with the drug are w/y and with the placebo x/z. The OR is the odds of improvement divided by the odds of no improvement. Odds ratios are notoriously difficult to interpret, but they are often quoted in papers so it is important to know how to calculate them. Detailed discussions of odds ratios can be found in the many critical review textbooks or on a variety of websites.

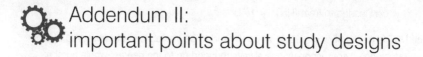

Addendum II: important points about study designs

Randomised, double-blind, placebo-controlled trial

An RCT is a study to investigate the effect of a treatment. There are at least two groups, one of which is given the experimental treatment and the other a placebo. The allocation of individuals to each of the groups is random. Double-blind means that neither the participant nor the doctor giving the treatment knows which group the patient is in.

Strengths

- Randomisation gives very similar groups and evenly distributes confounders.

- Double-blinding (ie doctors and patients unaware which treatment is given) minimises risk of biasing outcome.

- Use of control group allows clear comparisons to be made and minimises the influence of the placebo effect.

- RCTs are prospective, eliminating bias resulting from recall or recording of information.

- RCTs should use a standardised form for delivering the treatment (such as a blister pack for drugs or a clear protocol for psychological therapies) that minimises the chance of bias caused by variation in the way that the treatment is given.

Weaknesses

- Expensive

- Difficult to conduct

- Participants are a highly selected group and so less likely to be representative

- May identify statistically significant results that are not of clinical importance.

Important areas to think about

Randomisation

There are a number of different forms of randomisation (eg block randomisation, stratified randomisation). It is important to be aware of the differences between them and how they are conducted.

For randomisation to be most effective, the way in which the randomisation is done should not be open to influence by the researchers or anyone else involved. Methods such as computer-based randomisation are good; others (such as picking names from a hat) are more susceptible to bias.

Control groups

Control groups should always be as similar as possible to the study group. Any clear differences (eg using a control population of young students versus a study population of elderly men) will compromise the value of the study.

Ability to generalise

The study population should be comparable to the general population to whom the results might be applied. Again, a study on young students will probably be of little value when considering the best treatment for elderly men, however good the methodology may otherwise be. The inclusion and exclusion criteria used should be clearly stated.

Losses to follow-up

It is very unlikely that all the patients who begin the study will complete it successfully. Many will drop out for a variety of reasons, from logistical (eg moved away from the area) to clinical (eg unable to tolerate the drug given) to personal (eg simply decide they no longer wish to participate). There should be some mechanism for dealing with these cases, which should be explicitly stated. This might range from excluding their data altogether to including their last recorded data in the final analysis (known as 'last observation carried forward'), or even assuming that the outcome was the worst possible. These techniques are described as 'intention to treat' analyses, but you should always look for a fuller explanation of the methods if this phrase is used. It is not sufficient on its own to identify what has been done.

Outcome measures

It is clearly important to have a means of measuring outcome so that a judgement can be made about whether the intervention used was effective. The best measures are standardised and validated tools (eg the Beck Depression Inventory, Positive and Negative Symptoms of Schizophrenia scale), rather than subjective measures (eg asking the patient if he or she feels better).

Cohort study

A cohort is a group of individuals who share a common characteristic – such as living or working in a particular place, or having been exposed to a particular set of circumstances (eg taking a particular drug, exposure to asbestos). The purpose of a cohort study is to follow the group over time (ie a prospective study) to see what happens to the members of the cohort. These studies can be used to establish causation or simply to describe outcomes over time. They are also used to study a wide range of outcomes from a particular exposure.

Strengths

- Good for studying rare exposures
- Multiple outcomes can be studied from a single exposure
- Prospective design minimises errors as a result of recall or recording bias.

Weaknesses

- Expensive
- Resource intensive and difficult to carry out
- Only worthwhile in common diseases – otherwise cohort size needs to be very large
- May take many years for results to become clear
- Losses to follow-up may be heavy as a result of long timescale.

Important areas to think about

Criteria for selecting cohort

The means used for selecting members of the cohort needs to be clear. This may be straightforward (eg everyone born in a particular hospital on a particular day), but may require stricter definition (eg everyone exposed to more than a set level of radiation).

Outcomes

If a particular outcome is being looked for, again it must be clearly defined and the method of identifying it clearly stated. As far as possible the means of identifying outcomes should be standardised across the cohort.

Follow-up

Losses to follow-up are likely in a cohort study given the potentially long timescale, and the means of identifying and dealing with them must be clear. The impact upon the results needs to be considered, especially if the losses occur a long time in advance of the results being analysed.

Case–control study

A case–control study is essentially a comparison of individuals with and without a particular disorder, looking for previous exposure to a factor of interest. They are retrospective studies, and therefore involve looking back into the history of individuals who are currently known to suffer from the disorder of interest. The controls are selected with the aim of being as similar as possible to the cases except for the presence of the disorder. It is possible to 'match' cases and controls for potential confounding variables (such as age, sex, etc.), but doing so prevents examining the influence of these variables in the analysis.

Strengths

- Relatively cheap
- Straightforward to carry out
- Multiple exposures can be examined
- Rare diseases can be studied.

Weaknesses

- Retrospective nature risks bias (recall, information, recording)
- May be difficult to assemble control group
- Difficult to establish whether factor is linked to disease itself or to an aspect of the disease (eg severity of schizophrenia rather than presence of absence of schizophrenia)
- Difficult to establish temporal associations (ie did the exposure take place before or after the onset of the disease?)
- Cannot be used as evidence of causation.

Important points to think about

Bias

Bias is the biggest problem with case–control studies. This is largely a result of their retrospective nature. Recall bias involves those with an illness being more likely to remember possible causes; recording bias means that some events (eg obstetric complications) are more likely to be recorded than others (such as illicit drug use). Selection bias in identifying cases is also a problem, eg if hospital case registers are used, then this will exclude cases who did not reach hospital. In addition, those treated in hospital are likely to be different in terms of illness severity, etc. from those not treated in hospital. As a result, complex strategies may need to be devised to ensure that the case group is as representative as the general population of cases of the disorder in question as possible. Exam questions about case–control studies are very likely to ask about bias, so it is important to be aware of the potential sources and also of ways in which they might be combated.

Causation

Given the difficulties outlined above, a case–control study cannot be used to identify causation. Their value lies in identifying possible factors that may be responsible, and excluding those that are unlikely to be involved. Prospective studies such as cohort studies are able to provide much stronger evidence of causation.

5 Part II: the essay

What is an essay?

The word 'essay' can be traced to the French verb *essayer*, which means 'to attempt'. It was originally coined by the French writer, Michel de Montaigne, in 1580, to describe his collection of writings. The idea of an essay as 'an attempt' supports the underlying notion that an essay is not something that can be said to be right or wrong, but can be regarded as only an attempt to convey thoughts and ideas on a subject. Very often when approaching essays, candidates think of them very narrowly as an exercise in quoting as many facts as possible with an equally long list of references. However, the extensive amount of available writing on the subjects of essays generally agrees that the key point of an essay is that it is a treatment of a topic from the author's personal point of view.

The Royal College's view of the essay

The Royal College of Psychiatrists itself issues some basic guidance on the essay paper that all prospective candidates should read. This is available directly from the College, and can be found on their website in the 'Examination format' section (reached via the 'Training' link on the front page). It considers an essay to be:

> ... a short literary composition dealing with a subject informatively and logically in a legible prose style. It is not acceptable to submit merely a list of facts. The essay seeks not just factual information but the evaluation of this information. It is the one paper which requires candidates to use their judgement and to argue their case.

Breaking down this description leaves a number of key areas to address: legible prose style, evaluation of information and arguing the case.

Legible prose style

Legibility is clearly a vital component of any piece of writing. Increasingly in day-to-day life computers are revolutionising the appearance of most written work, but this luxury will not be available in the exam. Learning how to present a piece of writing well has useful application to daily practice as well to exam situations, and will bring rewards in both.

Handwriting is extremely variable and, although the bad reputation that doctors have acquired for their writing is largely unjustified, it can still be a problem for some. Most people are fully aware of how legible their handwriting is to others. It is important to be honest with yourself, and not be afraid to seek the opinions of others. If your colleagues have difficulty with your writing then it is likely that the examiners will as well. Problems in this area can very often be rectified by simple measures such as making writing larger and increasing the spacing between the words.

Allied to this, finding a pen that is comfortable to use and produces attractive text is invaluable. Cheap disposable ballpoints are to be found everywhere, but seldom produce attractive writing. They also tend to need to be pressed to the paper relatively hard, which can be very tiring, especially when (as in the exam) writing for long periods of time. Most stationery shops sell a wide variety of fibre-tip and rollerball pens that are a great improvement.

Presenting the essay well in other ways can also be of great benefit. Examiners marking the essay will see countless scripts in the course of the day, so any way of making the essay easy and pleasant to read is likely to produce an advantage. Although the exam regulations do not demand it, writing on alternate lines makes the text appear less dense and easier to follow. It has the added advantage of allowing small corrections or additions to be made at a later stage. The use of regular paragraph breaks (ideally with a blank line left between blocks of text) to mark the end of discussion of individual ideas provides an indication to the reader that a new idea is to be introduced and helps maintain the flow of the essay.

Finally, dividing the essay into sections and labelling these with subheadings will make the essay both easier to read and easier to write. Good planning at the outset is essential (see discussion below), and clear subheadings will make it obvious to the examiner what your structure is. Also, dividing the essay into sections allows you to tackle it one piece at a time, so the essay can be thought of as being composed of a number of 'mini-essays' which are written one at a time. Make sure that you give these sections meaningful names – examiners report seeing essays with sections entitled

'Main body', 'Point 1', etc. These are uninformative, and give the impression that you do not know what you are going to write about.

There are a number of means by which some candidates try to improve the presentation of their essays that will immediately annoy the examiner and should be avoided. These include the use of felt pens or coloured pens, underlining or highlighting of 'main points' and the use of 'bullet points' or long lists. Another common pitfall is 'margin drift', in which failure to begin each sentence at the leftmost margin leads to the body of the essay appearing to drift across the page:

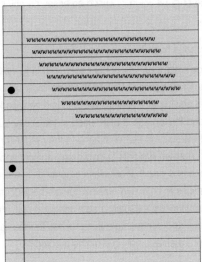

This looks sloppy and will not impress the examiner. Overall, your essay should appear as a professional document that would not look out of place in any other formal setting (such as a university exam, medical records, court of law).

Prose

An essay must be written as prose, ie in full sentences. This may seem obvious, but anecdotal reports from examiners reveal that some candidates present their essay in a 'bullet point' format or as lists of individual facts. Doing this makes it very difficult for the examiners to award marks. Also, you should avoid using the first person (eg 'in this essay I will try to demonstrate ...', 'I believe that ...'). Instead, use the third person (eg 'the aim of this essay is to ...', 'many are currently of the opinion that ...'), which once again gives the essay a professional feel.

Writing prose is a skill in itself, and although most junior psychiatrists will have written works of prose at either school or university, these skills will need to be revised and practised. It is a good idea to begin regularly to read articles both in the College journals (particularly the editorial or opinion columns) and also in non-medical publications such as quality newspapers (*The Times, Guardian, The Independent*, etc.). The aim is not to memorise the content of the articles but rather to gain an understanding of how the articles are constructed, and the techniques used by the writers to argue their case, synthesise information and arrive at a conclusion. Doing regular reading like this will also be of benefit in improving your general knowledge of current issues in psychiatry and the wider world, which will be of great value in writing an essay on any subject.

Evaluation of information

The second of the College's components of the essay relates to evaluating information. This involves closely examining a piece of information, considering points in favour of it and points against it, and arriving at a conclusion. This is otherwise known as critically discussing information, and this phrase is often used in the essay questions. The key point in the evaluation of evidence is demonstrating to the reader (or in this case the examiner) that you have considered points in favour and against and used this to arrive at a conclusion. This process is one that clinicians employ daily with all kinds of evidence, from journal articles to entries in nursing notes. The process of evaluating information in these circumstances is usually a subconscious one. However, in the exam it is necessary to be explicit and demonstrate this process to the examiner. It is similar to 'showing your working out' when attempting a maths problem.

Sources of information and evidence need to be thought about in broad terms. It is often assumed by candidates that only references to work published in medical journals are acceptable, but you must think more broadly than this. Reference can be made to (among many others) recent news items, Government policy, initiatives from the Royal College of Psychiatrists and events in day-to-day clinical practice. It is also perfectly acceptable to make direct references to your own experience for evidence such as a patient seen in clinic, a discussion at a ward round, a recent lecture or educational meeting. Other useful sources of 'evidence' are journals that collect together important or interesting articles (such as *Current Opinion in Psychiatry*), publications by the National Institute for Health and Clinical Excellence or NICE (all available on the NICE website) and local trust or hospital policy.

Remember that you must demonstrate awareness of important issues facing psychiatry and the medical profession, because appropriate references to these demonstrate knowledge of psychiatry that is not confined to textbooks. References to journals do have their place and, if you are able to include a reference to a relevant article, you will be given credit for it. However, rather than hoping that the subject of a particular article will come up as an essay, it is better to remember salient points of articles and find ways to include these in essays on related topics.

Arguing the case

As discussed above, the primary purpose of the essay is to produce a treatment of a particular topic from a personal point of view. It is therefore important at an early stage of planning the essay to consider what your response to the question is, and to structure the essay in such a way that it supports your point of view. As described above, it is necessary to consider alternative points of view and weigh up the pros and cons of each, but the overall direction of the essay should be to support your view on the subject.

Candidates are often wary of making statements of their own opinion, but including your own ideas and opinions in the essay not only makes it more interesting to read but also demonstrates your ability to think for yourself. It is also generally easier to make a convincing argument for a point of view that you hold yourself. One way of beginning to put your ideas together is to imagine that you are having a discussion with a friend or colleague on the subject in question, and consider what you would say and how you would support your argument. It may be helpful to reformulate the question as a statement, and then think about your response to it. For example, consider the question:

Describe how the presentation, assessment and treatment of schizophrenia differs in those with a learning disability compared with the general population.

This could be rephrased as a statement thus:

There is no difference in the presentation, assessment and treatment of schizophrenia between those with learning disabilities and the general population.

This statement should immediately provoke a response. You should consider whether you agree with the statement and why (or why not). Your response and the reasoning behind it can be used as the basis of the essay. It is quite reasonable to disagree strongly with the statement and say so, but you must be able to consider the evidence and support your argument accordingly. Almost any opinion can be legitimately expressed so long as it can be justified with reference to evidence, although great care must be taken with highly controversial or provocative opinions!

How the essay is marked

The essay is marked on four separate areas: content, coherence of argument, literacy and references. For each, a grade is given in one of six categories: excellent, pass, borderline pass, borderline fail, fail and very poor. An overall mark out of 10 is then given on the general impression of the essay and final decision about pass or fail made on that basis. The essay is scored overall in the same six categories.

To achieve a borderline pass (5/10) the essay needs to score at least a borderline pass in the literacy and coherence of argument sections, and similarly a borderline fail overall results from a borderline fail in the same two sections in the absence of exceptional scores elsewhere. Clearly, therefore, the literacy and coherence of argument components are favoured over the content and references components when making decisions about borderline cases. It is thus very important to make sure that, in preparation, attention is paid to the literacy (ie spelling, grammar, legibility, use of language). It is not difficult to get this right, and will immediately mark your essay out from many others and increase the chance of passing. Many candidates worry unduly about how many references they should include; in terms of passing the exam the literacy aspect is more important.

Preparation for the essay paper

As stated by the College and above, the essay is not primarily designed as a test of memory. There are no 'killer facts' or references for any particular topic that will guarantee an instant pass if included, or an instant fail if missed. Similarly, accurate quoting of a long list of references does not guarantee a high mark or even a pass.

The potential selection of subjects is very broad, and the chances of having prepared an essay on the specific topics that are asked are quite small. 'Question spotting' is notoriously unreliable – high-profile revision courses make regular efforts to guess the forthcoming topics, and are usually proved wrong. There is also much speculation on internet discussion boards about 'hot topics', but these are usually wrong as well. Occasionally recent articles from College journals (such as *Advances in Psychiatric Treatment*) have been used as the basis for questions, but this seems to be the exception rather than the rule.

Overall, relying on learning prepared essays or topics is a risky strategy. A much better approach is to learn and practise the skills of essay writing described above and combine these with a good general knowledge of clinical psychiatry and an awareness of important issues in the profession and beyond. It is reasonable to expect that anyone sitting the Part II exam has a sound knowledge of clinical practice and the theory underlying it. This knowledge tends to be static and can be derived from the standard texts and day-to-day work. However, equally important is to be well informed on current issues in psychiatry, mental health and healthcare provision in general. These are all likely to be relevant to any topic asked about, and appropriate reference to these issues demonstrates a broad knowledge of the area. The best way to gain such knowledge is to read widely, not only academic journals but also newspapers and magazines.

To give some examples, there are three broad areas of which it is important to have an understanding: issues in the media, issues in the Royal College of Psychiatrists and Government policy.

Mental health is an issue that is of great concern to the public, and almost every day there are items in the news that have some relevance, eg there is considerable debate in the media at present about the risks posed by people with mental illness. Internet sites such as BBC News have sections devoted to health, which are a good place to start. Most quality newspapers also have websites with a lot of useful content. Listening to the radio (especially the current affairs programmes on Radio 4) on the way to and from work can also provide a great deal of useful material, and can help you to think about the arguments surrounding these issues.

The Royal College of Psychiatrists regularly launches new initiatives and its website contains much useful information. Being able to make reference to resources provided by the College in essays looks good – after all, it is the body of which you are trying to become a member. For example, the recent 'Partners in Care' initiative heavily promoted the role of carers in mental illness and provided considerable resources for them.

Finally, Government policy with regard to the NHS and mental health services in particular is ever changing and has considerable implications for how psychiatry is practised. Often the views of psychiatrists do not accord with the views of the Government, and this conflict can pose many problems. Recent issues include the proposals for the new Mental Health Act and the establishment of NICE with the subsequent debate on the role of guidelines. Also, the National Service Framework for Mental Health contains much of relevance, and knowledge of the basic principles is very helpful.

Types of question

The exam paper consists of three questions. There are noticeable similarities in the way that the questions are formed, although clearly the subject matter varies considerably. In the past it was generally accepted that there would be one question on general psychiatry, one on one of the main specialities (child, forensic, etc.) and a third on general aspects of psychiatry. In recent times this appears to have changed, and it is increasingly difficult to predict the subject area for the questions.

There are exceptions, but reviewing past essay papers reveals three basic types of question: discussion of a general statement, comparison of two related subjects and discussion related to a specific diagnosis.

Discussion of a general statement

This type of question consists of a statement that is to be critically discussed. The statement itself is generally a fairly broad one, but often it is required that reference be made to a particular diagnosis. An example of such a question might be:

> 'The legacy of psychiatry in the early twenty-first century will be that it was the era in which the hospitals were closed and the prisons expanded.' Discuss this statement critically with reference to appropriate evidence.

Note that 'appropriate evidence' does not necessarily include (and certainly is not limited to) articles published in scientific journals. What constitutes 'evidence' is discussed above. Simple statements such as these are often quite broad, and may not be directly related to a specific illness at all. Although these may be thought of as vague, they also place few restrictions upon your answer.

Another example that refers to a specific diagnosis might be:

> 'The recent downgrading in classification of cannabis means that there is no cause for concern regarding its use by patients with mental illness.' Discuss this statement critically with reference to schizophrenia.

The answer should take the form of a general discussion, with reference to schizophrenia for illustration. It is important not to be distracted into a discussion of schizophrenia primarily, but to stick to the substance of the statement.

Questions such as these are perhaps the easiest to score highly in, because they do not necessarily require specialist knowledge. Either of the two questions above could be answered by an informed layperson, and the examiners will be looking for a broad view of the subject.

Comparison of two related subjects

This type of question involves a consideration of the difference between two separate quantities. These questions can be quite broad ranging, and the comparison may be between anything such as the presentation and treatment of two diseases, or the relative advantages and disadvantages of particular models of service delivery. An example of such a question might be:

'How does the presentation, assessment and management of schizophrenia differ in those with learning disability compared with the general adult population? What are the consequences of these differences for service provision?'

When approaching a comparison question, it is important not simply to describe each of the two themes independently. Although description is important, an effort must be made to compare the two actively by considering which aspects are the same and which differ, and to draw conclusions from these differences and similarities. This can be done either point by point, or else by first describing the two and then highlighting the important areas. You may wish to practise both styles of answer to see which one you are more comfortable with.

Discussion related to a specific diagnosis

This type of question is centred around a specific diagnosis, and to attempt such a question it is necessary to have some knowledge of the disorder in question. It may be a simple subject such as the management of a condition or a more complex issue related to the diagnosis in question. A simple discussion might be:

'Discuss the management options for treatment-resistant depression and outline the likely prognosis in each case.'

A more complex question might be framed thus:

'Discuss drug treatments and psychological therapies involved in treating borderline personality disorder, and outline how these might be implemented in practice.'

Dissecting the question

Each question consists of a number of components, and so careful reading of the question and subsequent addressing of every point is vital in order to maximise your mark. If you do not do so, then immediately the number of marks available for the essay as a whole is reduced. To be sure that all points have been addressed, it is important to dissect the question thoroughly before attempting it. It has been said (and this is also true for patient management problems) that not a word of the question is wasted – so attention must be given to all of them. For example, consider the following question:

> 'Antipsychotic medication has no role in the treatment of personality disorders.' Discuss this statement critically with reference to the range of possible treatments and their theoretical basis.

This question has three separate components, all of which need to be considered: critical discussion of the statement, discussion of the range of the treatments and for each brief discussion of its theoretical basis. All these points must be addressed in the essay, so it is important to incorporate them all into the essay plan.

The principles of critical discussion have already been outlined above, but in this particular situation it will be necessary to consider the statement and its implications, and outline your response to it. Second, addressing the range of treatments clearly implies that reference will need to be made to several different treatments, rather than just one. It might be tempting from the way in which the question is framed to write only about antipsychotics, but to maximise the opportunities for gaining marks the role of other treatments (biological, psychological and social) will need to be considered as well. Finally, having discussed the range it is necessary to pay attention to the theoretical basis for each of the treatments discussed.

Even though you may feel that you have very limited knowledge, it is still important to attempt each section of the question. Although you may not be able to quote specific papers or studies concerning (as in this case) the theoretical basis for drugs in personality disorder, your general knowledge on the mode of action of the drugs and of the presentation of those with personality disorder should enable you to make some general statements about how they might work. Clearly, in order to gain the highest marks a good knowledge of the literature will be required, but unless you attempt that section of the question in some form you will not be able to gain any marks for it.

On the day

The essay paper is the second of the morning papers, after the critical review.

Choosing the right question

The essay paper lasts for 90 minutes, which is actually much more than is required to write a suitable essay. There is therefore plenty of time to think about which question you are going to do. There is no rush to choose a question, and if you decide in haste you may regret it after 40 minutes when you have run out of things to say and there is not sufficient time adequately to attempt another question. It is all too easy to panic as people around you begin to write frenziedly within the first few minutes of the exam. Do not allow yourself to be rushed into starting in an attempt to keep up – those who start quickly very often finish quickly (and prematurely) because they have not thought their essay through properly.

As discussed above, no matter how much you have prepared there is a good chance that you will not have specifically revised any of the questions with which you are faced. If there is a question that you have specifically revised and are happy with, then the decision is an easy one but otherwise (and perhaps more likely) you will need to consider for which question you can write the best answer. Your immediate response to the lack of 'hot topics' will probably be feelings of gloom and despondency (eg 'I can't answer any of these, I haven't revised them!'), but you should ignore these and instead think carefully about the questions that you are presented with. For each, begin to dissect it into its component parts as described above and consider how you might approach these. It may help to jot down some of your thoughts for each and rough out a basic structure. Once you have done this, it should become clear which of the three questions you are best equipped to approach.

It is important at this stage to take your time – with the right question and a good plan (and depending on how fast you write) an adequate essay can be written in about 60 minutes. However, this will differ from person to person and in your preparation practising essays under timed conditions should give you a good idea of how long you are likely to need.

Planning the essay

Once you have decided on a question, constructing an essay plan is the next step. This is the key to your essay, and getting it right will make writing the essay itself very much easier. Everyone has his or her own approach to writing essay plans (and therefore to essays), but a commonly described model for planning an essay is the 'five paragraph' approach. This consists of an introduction and conclusion with three points covered in the three middle paragraphs. In the context of the essays for the MRCPsych exam it may be more appropriate to think in terms of sections rather than paragraphs (because you will need more than one paragraph per section), and clearly there may be more or fewer than three main points.

In choosing the question, you will have already begun to think about your response, and the purpose of the plan is briefly to write down your ideas with some additional structure. For each of the sections (introduction, conclusion and main points) make brief notes of your main ideas and also any factual information that you want to include (such as incidence and prevalence rates, definitions) that you can refer back to later. Write the plan in short phrases and words that will prompt you as you write the essay itself. The plan should be written in such a way that writing the essay itself is mainly a question of 'fleshing out' the phrases in your plan. By the time you have finished your plan, you should have a clear idea of the points and arguments that you are going to use and the order in which you are going to do so. This will give you confidence when it comes to writing the essay itself.

An important part of preparation for the exam is practising how to write plans. This is generally much quicker than practising writing many essays and it will also closely mimic the experience of being in the exam. It is much easier to write a good essay from a well thought-out plan than to make it up as you go along. Opinion is divided concerning whether you should leave your plan for the examiner's inspection. Some will say that the examiner will see from your plan the direction in which you are taking the essay and give you some credit for it, even if you are unable to finish. Others say that examiners will give marks only on the basis of the written essay, and the plan is irrelevant. The College view (as stated by examiners) is that the plan can be written at the start but must be crossed out (one line is sufficient). This has the advantage that, although the plan is clearly not part of the essay, the examiner can still read it.

Constructing the essay

The first section is the introduction to the essay. The introduction should begin with general points concerning the subject under discussion that set the scene for the essay. It is helpful to include basic factual information, such as definitions of the terms to be used, demographic data. The introduction should also contain a short statement of your response to the question, which is referred to as the 'thesis statement'. This can include your comments or criticisms of the questions (eg 'this is an outrageous assertion' or 'this is a highly controversial area'). It may also be useful to define any terms used in the questions (eg 'schizophrenia is defined in the ICD-10 as …', 'amitriptyline is an antidepressant drug, belonging to the group known as tricyclic antidepressants on account of their chemical structure'). Following the thesis statement, the various points or arguments to be addressed in the rest of the essay should be listed, ideally in order of their importance or relative strength of argument. Ideally, the introduction should conclude with a sentence or sentences that introduce the first point.

Each of the main points should be addressed in its own section. Using subheadings to separate these sections makes it clear both to the examiners and to yourself where each starts and finishes, and gives some additional structure which is helpful when writing. The basic structure, irrespective of the point being made, is the same for each. The section should begin with a short statement of the essential feature of the point, followed by a more detailed discussion of the points that you wish to use in support of this statement. The discussion should be kept firmly focused on the subject of the section, and all the points mentioned should be relevant to it. There are no specific rules about how many sections there should be (or indeed how long the essay is overall), but a thorough discussion of a small number of important points is likely to be easier to follow and have greater impact than skimming over a large number of points.

Finally, the aim of the final section (or conclusion) is to pull together the thesis statement from the introduction and the important aspects of each of the subsections. General points can also be made about the implications of the discussion and suggestions made about which future developments would be useful or important. The conclusion should leave the reader with a clear impression of your overall response to the essay. It is best not to introduce very much new material in the conclusion, but instead to restate concisely what has already been discussed in the previous sections. It is wise to avoid using clichés or 'stock phrases' such as 'Further research is needed in this area' or 'This is a challenging area of psychiatry'. If you feel that such points are important, make sure that you enlarge on this statement with your ideas, eg if more research is required make some suggestions about what particular aspects of the topic should be researched and how this might be carried out.

The overall view of the essay can be summarised by the well-worn (but still very helpful) phrase 'Tell them what you're going to tell them, tell them, then tell them what you've told them'. The introduction briefly lists the points, the main body discusses them in detail and the conclusion summarises them. Following this format makes your point several times over, and will communicate your point of view efficiently and leave the examiner impressed with the clarity and coherence of your argument.

Conclusion

Although initially a daunting prospect, the essay paper is the one area of the exam where you have the opportunity to express yourself freely and demonstrate your knowledge and skills. Thorough preparation is essential, but spending time developing skills in writing rather than trying to memorise large quantities of factual information will equip you to tackle most of the questions that you are likely to face. As stated at the start of this chapter, an essay is primarily about putting forward a personal point of view on a topic. It is vital to include your own ideas and opinions, and failing to do so is to miss the point of the paper entirely.

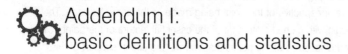 # Addendum I: basic definitions and statistics

Sources of information

There are a number of different sources of information regarding incidence and prevalence data. These are listed below, and are referred to by abbreviations (given in brackets) throughout. This list is provided for reference only, and more detailed reading of the sources listed is strongly recommended. Most of these resources are available on the internet, and can easily be located by searching for the titles given below.

WHO. *The ICD-10 Classification of Mental and Behavioural Disorders*, 10th revision. Geneva: World Health Organization, 1992. (ICD-10)

APA. *The Diagnostic and Statistical Manual of Mental Disorders*, 4th edn. Chicago: American Psychiatric Association, 1992. (DSM-IV)

Singleton et al. *Psychiatric Morbidity Among Adults Living in Private Households*. London: Office for National Statistics, 2000. (PMAALPH)

Mental Health: A Report of the Surgeon General. Washington DC: US Department of Health and Human Services, 1999. (USSG)

National Epidemiologic Survey on Alcohol and Related Conditions, 2001–2002. (NESARC)

Appleby et al. *Safety First, Report of the National Confidential Inquiry into Suicide and Homicide by People with Mental Illness*. London: The Stationery Office, 2001 (NCIS).

Depression

- A disorder of affect characterised by low mood, loss of interest and enjoyment and reduced energy leading to increased fatigability and diminished activity (ICD-10)
- Lifetime prevalence 16%, point prevalence 26 per 1000 (PMAALPH)
- Prevalence of depressive episode 6.5%, unipolar depression 5.3% (USSG).

Bipolar affective disorder

- A disorder characterised by repeated episodes in which the patient's mood and activity levels are significantly disturbed, this disturbance consisting on some occasions of an elevation of mood and increased energy and activity (mania) and on others of a lowering of mood and decreased energy and activity (depression) (ICD-10)
- Bipolar I disorder or BP-I (episode of mania) or bipolar II disorder or BP-II (episode of hypomania plus depression) (DSM-IV)
- Prevalence of BP-I: 1.1% (USSG)
- Prevalence of BP-II: 0.6% (USSG).

Generalised anxiety disorder

- Anxiety that is generalised and persistent but not restricted to or strongly predominating in any particular environmental circumstances (ICD-10)
- Prevalence 44 per 1000 (PMAALP) or 2.4% (USSG).

Panic disorder

- Recurrent attacks of severe anxiety (panic) that are not restricted to any particular situation or set of circumstances, and that are therefore unpredictable (ICD-10)
- Prevalence 1.6% (USSG).

Obsessive–compulsive disorder

- Recurrent obsessional thoughts or compulsive acts
- Obsessional thoughts are ideas, images or impulses that enter the individual's mind again and again in a stereotyped form
- Compulsive acts or rituals are stereotyped behaviours that are repeated again and again
- Prevalence 11 per 1000 (PMAALP) or 2.4% (USSG).

Post-traumatic stress disorder

- Arises as a delayed and/or protracted response to a stressful event or situation (either short or long lasting) of an exceptionally threatening or catastrophic nature, which is likely to cause pervasive distress in almost anyone (ICD-10)
- Prevalence 3.6% (USSG).

Schizophrenia

- Disorders characterised by fundamental and characteristic distortions of thinking and perception, and by inappropriate or blunted affect (ICD-10)
- Prevalence 1.3% (USSG).

Personality disorder

- A severe disturbance in the characterological constitution and behavioural tendencies of the individual, usually involving several areas of personality and almost always associated with considerable personal and social disruption (ICD-10)
- Prevalence (all types) 14.8% (NESARC).

The following breakdown (also from NESARC) refers to personality disorder as defined in DSM-IV:

Obsessive–compulsive	7.9%
Paranoid	4.4%
Antisocial	3.6%
Schizoid	3.1%
Avoidant	2.4%
Histrionic	1.8%
Dependent	0.5%

Suicide

- A wilful, self-inflicted, life-threatening act resulting in death'
- Prevalence: 6000 per year in UK
- 25% in contact with mental health services in the year before death
- 23% within 3 months of discharge, most in 1–2 weeks post discharge
- 16% were psychiatric inpatients, 25% died in the first week after admission (NCIS).

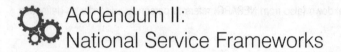 # Addendum II:
National Service Frameworks

National Service Framework for Mental Health (Department of Health, 1999)

Standard 1: Mental Health Promotion
Health and social services should:

Promote mental health for all, working with individuals and communities.

Combat discrimination against individuals and groups with mental health problems, and promote their social inclusion.

Standard 2: Primary Care and Access to Services
Any service user who contacts their primary healthcare team with a common mental health problem should:

Have their mental health needs identified and assessed.

Be offered effective treatments, including referral to specialist services for further assessment, treatment and care if they require it.

Standard 3: Primary Care and Access to Services
Any individual with a common mental health problem should:

Be able to make contact around the clock with the local services necessary to meet their needs and receive adequate care.

Be able to use NHS Direct, as it develops, for first-level advice and referral on to specialist helplines or to local services.

Standard 4: Effective Services for People with Severe Mental Illness
All mental health service users on the Care Programme Approach (CPA) should:

Receive care that optimises engagement, prevents or anticipates crisis, and reduces risk.

Have a copy of a written care plan that:

- includes the action to be taken in a crisis by service users, their carers and their care coordinators

- advises GPs how they should respond if service users need additional help

- is regularly reviewed by the care coordinator.

Be able to access services 24 hours a day, 365 days a year

Standard 5: Effective Services for People with Severe Mental Illness

Each service user who is assessed as requiring a period of care away from home should have:

Timely access to an appropriate hospital bed or alternative bed or place that is:

- in the least restrictive environment consistent with the need to protect them and the public

- as close to home as possible.

A copy of a written after-care plan agreed on discharge, which sets out the care and rehabilitation to be provided, identifies the care coordinator and specifies the action to be taken in a crisis.

Standard 6: Caring about Carers

All individuals who provide regular and substantial care for a person on the CPA should:

Have an assessment of their caring, physical and mental health needs, repeated on at least an annual basis.

Have their own written care plan, which is given to them and implemented in discussion with them.

Standard 7: Preventing Suicide

Local health and social care communities should prevent suicides by:

Promoting mental health for all, working with individuals and communities (Standard 1).

Delivering high-quality primary mental health care (Standard 2).

Ensuring that anyone with a mental health problem can contact local services via the primary care team, a helpline or an A&E department (Standard 3).

Ensuring that individuals with severe and enduring mental illness have a care plan that meets their specific needs, including access to services round the clock (Standard 4).

Providing safe hospital accommodation for individuals who need it (Standard 5).

Enabling individuals caring for someone with severe mental illness to receive the support that they need to continue to care (Standard 6).

In addition:

Supporting local prison staff in preventing suicides among prisoners.

Ensuring that staff are competent to assess the risk of suicide among individuals at greatest risk.

Developing local systems for suicide audit to learn lessons and take any necessary action.

National Service Framework for Older People (Department of Health 2001)

Standard 1: Rooting Out Age Discrimination

NHS services will be provided, regardless of age, on the basis of clinical need alone.

Social care services will not use age in their eligibility criteria or policies, to restrict access to available services.

Standard 2: Person-centred Care

NHS and social care services treat older people as individuals and enable them to make choices about their own care. This is achieved through the single assessment process, integrated commissioning arrangements and integrated provision of services, including community equipment and continence services.

Standard 3: Intermediate Care

Older people will have access to a new range of intermediate care services at home or in designated care settings, to promote their independence by providing enhanced services from the NHS and councils to prevent unnecessary hospital admission and effective rehabilitation services to enable early discharge from hospital and to prevent premature or unnecessary admission to long-term residential care.

Standard 4: General Hospital Care

Older people's care in hospital is delivered through appropriate specialist care and by hospital staff who have the right set of skills to meet their needs.

Standard 5: Stroke

The NHS will take action to prevent strokes, working in partnership with other agencies where appropriate.

People who are thought to have had a stroke have access to diagnostic services, are treated appropriately by a specialist stroke service, and subsequently, with their carers, participate in a multidisciplinary programme of secondary prevention and rehabilitation.

Standard 6: Falls

The NHS, working in partnership with councils, takes action to prevent falls and reduce resultant fractures or other injuries in their populations of older people. Older people who have fallen receive effective treatment and, with their carers, receive advice on prevention through a specialised falls service.

Standard 7: Mental Health in Older People

Older people who have mental health problems have access to integrated mental health services, provided by the NHS and councils to ensure effective diagnosis, treatment and support, for them and for their carers.

Standard 8: The Promotion of Health and Active Life in Older Age

The health and well-being of older people is promoted through a coordinated programme of action led by the NHS with support from councils.

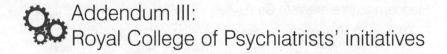

Addendum III:
Royal College of Psychiatrists' initiatives

Defeat Depression (January 1992–December 1996)

The 'Defeat Depression' campaign was launched in January 1992 and ran for 5 years. The campaign had three stated aims:

To educate health professionals, particularly general practitioners, about recognition and management of depression.

To educate the general public about depression and the availability of treatment. In order to encourage people to seek help earlier.

To reduce the stigma associated with depression.

RCPsych (1992)

The College established two committees (a Management Committee and a Scientific Advisory Committee) to run the campaign and to provide appropriate advice. A variety of measures were used to meet the aims, and by the end of the campaign it was reported to have had 'many successes', the extent of which was documented and published.

One activity was the production of a range of leaflets dealing with depression in all populations (including old age, learning disability, etc.) and addressing a variety of other issues relevant to depression (such as alcohol abuse, effect of depression in the workplace). These are still available from the College website (www.rcpsych.ac.uk).

Changing Minds (October 1998–October 2003)

The 'Changing Minds' campaign was launched in October 1998 with a clear agenda to address the problems of stigmatisation of people with mental health problems. The College sees public education as one of its main objectives, and felt that after the success of 'Defeat Depression' it should focus upon stigma associated with mental illness more generally.

The campaign was aimed at addressing stigma in anxiety, depression, schizophrenia, dementia, alcohol and drug addiction, and eating disorders. The target populations included doctors, children and young people, employers, the media and the general public. The campaign aimed to 'increase public and professional understanding of mental health problems and to reduce stigma and discrimination'.

Over the time that the campaign operated, a large amount of material was created and assembled into a 'toolkit' which was made available on the campaign website (www.changingminds.co.uk); a separate site dealing more academically with the subject was also launched (www.stigma.org). Although the campaign has now formally closed, the College announced their intention of continuing to develop and distribute the materials, and acknowledged that despite the campaign 'tackling the stigma of mental illness is an enduring task'.

2001: A Mind Odyssey (July 2001–June 2002)

'2001: A Mind Odyssey' was a short initiative organised by the College in 2001 to highlight the links of the arts, the mind and psychiatry. The campaign aimed to increase awareness among staff and patients of the potential therapeutic benefits of artistic expression, and to encourage people to explore their own creativity further.

The initiative ran over the course of 1 year and a number of events were held as a part of it. One highlight was a 3-day film festival in which a number of important films (including 'Iris') with a connection to psychiatry were shown. There were also a number of art exhibitions and other seminars held under the auspices of the campaign.

It was officially closed at the 2002 College Annual Meeting.

Partners in Care (January 2004–June 2005)

'Partners in Care' was launched as a joint initiative between the College and the Princess Royal Trust for Carers. It was initially intended to run for 1 year, but this was later extended to 18 months with the campaign coming to an official end in June 2005. The initiative was championed by the President at the time (Dr Mike Shooter), who had a particular interest in this area. He commented at the launch of the campaign 'The carer's voice in decision making about admission and discharge is ignored at everyone's peril – and yet it so often is'.

The aims of the campaign were to:

Highlight the problems faced by carers of all ages of people with different mental health problems and learning disabilities

Encourage true partnerships between carers, patients and professionals

RCPsych (2004)

The campaign placed emphasis on the following points:

Carers play a vital role in looking after, and promoting the wellbeing of people with mental health problems – carers' responsibilities need greater recognition.

Carers themselves can suffer from mental health problems, often because of a lack of support.

Specialist help is available for carers of someone with a mental health problem.

A number of activities were commenced as part of the campaign, including the production of a range of materials (leaflets, booklets, videos and CD-ROMs), promotion of the subject in the media, specific training of professionals, etc.

The campaign was officially closed in June 2005.

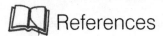 References

Defeat depression

See www.rcpsych.ac.uk/campaigns/defeatdepression.aspx

Paykel ES et al. The Defeat Depression Campaign: pyschiatry in the public arena. *American Journal of Psychiatry* 1997, 154, (festscrift supplement): 59–65.

Paykel ES et al. Changes in public attitudes to depression during the Defeat Depression Campaign. *British Journal of Psychiatry* 1998; 173: 519–522.

Partners in Care

See also www.rcpysch.ac.uk/campaigns/partnersincare.aspx

Shooter M. Partners in Care – who cares for the carers? *Pyschiatric Bulletin* 2004; 28: 313–314.

6 Sample essays

This chapter contains example essay questions and answers, covering a range of both general and speciality topics. These essays have been written in line with the principles outlined above. Several of the questions given below are very similar to those that have appeared in the exam in the past. As stated previously, it is notoriously difficult to predict which subjects will appear, and the choice of subjects in these essays does not represent any attempt to predict future questions.

You should use this chapter to familiarise yourself with the types of question asked, and the ways in which these questions can be approached. You may wish to try answering the questions yourself under exam conditions. However, it is important to remember that there is no right or wrong answer to an essay – these examples show just one way of answering each question. A well-constructed essay arguing the complete opposite would score just as highly. Any of the essays here would gain very high marks in the exam – although you should aspire to this, it is not necessary to produce a very high-quality essay in order to pass!

A list of references to papers and publications is provided at the end of each essay, although in the real exam it is sufficient simply to name the authors and date of the paper that you are referencing in the text. Some of these essays have fewer references than others, and some have none at all. As has been discussed earlier, making reference to evidence is much broader than using journal articles alone. All of these essays make reference to a range of evidence from a range of sources.

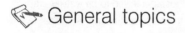 General topics

Essay 1

'Work-related stress is the biggest occupational health problem facing modern society. Discuss the factors that lead up to this.'

Introduction

Stress has been defined by the Health and Safety Executive as 'the adverse reaction people have to excessive pressures or other types of demand placed upon them', and this reaction can consist of physical, psychological and social difficulties. Stress directly attributable to occupation ('work-related stress') is an increasing and very important problem that poses many challenges to society. The pressures of modern life have led to increased pressure to perform at work, and the demands of work have also increased. Over recent years, awareness of the problems caused by stress has increased but little has been done to combat it.

There are a variety of causes of work-related stress and also reasons why it has become such a problem. They can be briefly summarised in terms of change and ignorance. First, there have been changes in society that have led to increased expectations of individuals to work. Second, and as a result of this, there have been changes in working practices that have conspired to increase demands placed on individuals. These problems have been compounded by ignorance of the problems caused by stress – an ignorance that is seen in the general public and also in the corporate structures themselves and even among psychiatrists.

The aim of this essay is to discuss these causes and in doing so to propose some ways in which the problems might be addressed.

Changes in society and culture of work

Recent years have witnessed a considerable change in the way in which the world of work operates. In the heyday of the manufacturing industries in the UK, most people could expect little difficulty in finding work and the promise of a 'job for life' when they did so. Over time, this picture has changed dramatically and currently most people expect to work in a number of different jobs over time, which may be in a variety of different areas. Retraining is commonplace, and there is often a great deal of competition to gain desirable jobs, and also to keep them once appointed. Many businesses operate a 'pyramid structure' whereby those perceived to be weaker are shed at regular intervals, with only those best able to compete surviving. At the same time, changes in society have led to an increased expectation of standard of living, with most people owning their own home and car, taking foreign holidays, etc. Society tends to appraise and judge people in terms of how much they earn and measure their degree of achievement accordingly. Pressure is on those of all ages to dress in the latest style. All these things bring with them associated costs and to service a 'modern-day' lifestyle can be very expensive.

The role of women in the workplace is also changing, such that many more women work in increasingly senior roles. It is also commonplace for women with young families to return to work early rather than look after the children (as was the 'traditional' role). As described above, the need for increased income to maintain a particular lifestyle is another motivator for women to return to work.

These factors together have led to a very pressured and stressful working environment. In many jobs, employees are under constant pressure to improve and produce better work in shorter periods of time. Working hours have increased and, despite the best efforts of various pieces of legislation (such as the European Working Time Directive or EWTD), working hours in the UK are among the longest in Europe. Such long hours disrupt family life, and the alternatives (such as shift work patterns) are unattractive to many. Medicine is not exempt, although traditionally working hours have been longer than they are at present. However, fitting medical rotas into the EWTD has resulted in wholesale adaptation of shift work that is unpopular because it results in regular periods of disrupted hours.

All these aspects conspire to place large amounts of stress on individuals. Not only is there great pressure at work, but traditional means for relaxing (such as spending time with friends and family, pursuing hobbies) are increasingly denied as a result of shortage of time and exhaustion. This can in turn lead to mental illnesses such as anxiety or depression which carry with them additional difficulties.

The impact of this on society cannot be underestimated. Days taken off work as a result of sickness cost businesses and society greatly, and also the businesses are unlikely to get the best performance from an overstretched workforce. Some professions in particular (eg nursing) are suffering recruitment crises as a result of unhealthy working practices and perceived low pay.

Overall, the significant changes seen in society and in the culture of work have contributed greatly to the current levels of stress. However, the response to these changes has often not been as robust as it could have been, often as a result of ignorance.

Ignorance of the general public

Awareness of mental health issues in the general public is known to be poor. The Royal College of Psychiatrists has made numerous valiant efforts to increase awareness (such as the Changing Minds campaign) but it is not clear how much impact they have had. Sensational coverage in the media of occasions when things go wrong serves only to increase stigma and stifle sensible information giving. Mental illness of all kinds often goes unrecognised and comes to professional attention only when a crisis is reached.

The same ignorance unfortunately applies to the problems of stress in the workplace.

People are often slow to recognise the signs of stress in themselves and to take appropriate action. Men in particular are often reluctant to admit how they are feeling, especially to admit to difficulties in coping with a specific situation. This may be in part because it is perceived as failure or weakness to admit that one is having difficulties, and the action involved (such as looking for a different job, or accepting a less responsible and hence a lower-paid position) may be unpalatable. This is compounded if the employer is unsympathetic.

Second, friends and family of the person affected may be unaware of the problems and unaware of how they may present. This again may lead to a delay in the problems being recognised and addressed.

Informing the general public about all mental health issues is very important, and in particular attention needs to be drawn to the problems of work-related stress. However, also of great importance is advice to the employers on their own role and responsibilities in this area.

Ignorance of employers

As described above, the change in working practices in the UK has contributed largely to the increased levels of stress at work. In particular, the high-pressure methods of employers and the uncertainty of retaining employment are significant. These problems are often compounded by the apparent ignorance of many companies of the importance of maintaining a healthy workforce. A workforce containing overstretched, stressed individuals is likely overall to be less productive and cost the company more, even though it may require a reduction in overall hours, a change in working practices and investment in the workforce. Some companies (such as Google and Apple) pride themselves on treating their employees well, and they have constructed impressive 'campus' environments. Although the demands placed on the employees may still be great, the flexible working practices and pleasant environment are likely to extract the best from the workforce. The success and popularity of these companies among employees is undisputed.

It is the role of the occupational health department in any large company to consider the health of the employees, but they are often not proactive in terms of health promotion. Work-related stress needs to be recognised as an important problem and measures need to be taken by such departments to promote the health of their employees.

Ignorance of psychiatrists

There are two ways in which the ignorance of psychiatrists contributes to the overall burden of work-related stress.

First, people referred to psychiatric outpatient clinics may be suffering from problems related to work but this may not always be elicited in the history. For the reasons given above, people may be reluctant to attribute their difficulties to stress at work and so, unless specifically asked about (and sometimes even then!), it may be missed. The 'occupational history' section of the personal history is often skimmed over, but it remains a very important component that should not be neglected. If work-related stress is missed as a significant contributor, the presented problems may prove difficult to treat. It is therefore very important that the role of stress at work should be recognised by psychiatrists and routinely considered in outpatient assessments.

Second, psychiatrists are likely to be just as guilty of ignorance of their own work-related difficulties. Consultant psychiatrists bear considerable responsibility and working conditions are often worse than they should be. There are many demands on a consultant's time and important decisions are constantly being made. It is very important that psychiatrists are aware of their own levels of stress, and take appropriate action if they become too high. Similarly, all those working in this area need to be aware of the possibility of excessive stress in colleagues.

Once again, a partial answer to this problem is to increase education and training of psychiatrists in managing the problems caused by stress at work. The management of these problems is likely to involve all members of the multidisciplinary team, and psychological interventions can be of particular benefit in teaching coping strategies and methods of avoiding stress.

Conclusion

Work-related stress is a complicated problem, and contributory factors arise from a number of sources. A change in the culture of work over time has increased demands placed on employees, and society demands an ever-increasing standard of living for people to feel valued and accepted. These problems have been compounded by the ignorance of the general public, employers and mental health services.

For this problem to be addressed it is necessary to have thorough education of all concerned, and to follow certain examples of work environments that are conducive to good health as well as to productivity. Friends, families and mental health services should be confident in their response to difficulties when they arise, and prompt help should be available. Research is required into the ways in which stress may affect individuals and into what treatment modalities are most successful.

There are no quick or easy solutions to these problems, but by working together as individuals – employees, employers and psychiatrists – progress will be made in addressing this challenging area.

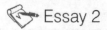 Essay 2

'Discuss the relationship between homelessness and mental illness, and outline potential solutions to the difficulties posed.'

Introduction

Homelessness is a significant problem in the UK that goes largely unrecognised and is underestimated. A person can be described as homeless if he or she has no fixed address or permanent place of residence. Although most people might consider homeless individuals to be those sleeping rough, this accounts for a small proportion of the true figure. Approximately 500 people sleep rough on any given night, of whom about half are in London. However, according to the charity Crisis there are 380 000 people in total who are homeless, including squatters, those living in bed and breakfast establishments and those in hostels. Homeless people are therefore a large and diverse population who have similarly varied needs.

It is important that psychiatrists are aware of homeless individuals, because having a mental illness increases the chances of subsequently becoming homeless and being homeless increases the risk of having a mental illness. Schizophrenia, affective disorders and substance misuse are all increased in this population (Scott, 1993). As in many areas, Tudor Hart's (1971) 'inverse care law' applies, such that those in greatest need have the greatest difficult in accessing the services that they need. Homeless people are a vulnerable group by virtue of their status.

The aim of this essay is to outline some of the difficulties posed in the care of homeless people and to outline how these might be addressed.

Access to services

The first problem that homeless people face with regard to mental health care (or indeed health care of any kind) is that of access. The lack of a fixed abode largely precludes the normal mechanisms for accessing health care. GPs may refuse to register a patient with no fixed address, and health authorities are generally reluctant to take responsibility for someone who cannot be proved to 'belong' to them. Being deprived access to primary care similarly restricts access to secondary care, and individuals will become dependent upon opportunist access via the A&E department. This brings its own difficulties, because there is a lack of continuity of care and also less opportunity for long-term follow-up. Similarly, there may not be the opportunities to obtain repeat prescriptions, etc.

Children of homeless people are impacted on in a similar way. They are less likely to attend school regularly, and so they are deprived not only of education but also of the opportunities for health care that school provides. They may miss out on immunisations, etc., and signs of mental illness may not be picked up. The impact of untreated mental illness on their education and future prospects is potentially severe.

Extent of current provision

It is not always easy to establish who is responsible for the care of homeless people. In most areas, responsibility is determined by address and so in the absence of an address the situation becomes much more complex. There are a number of statutory bodies that can be said to have a role in dealing with homeless people, and these include Social Services, local authority housing departments, hospital emergency services and the police. However, there are also a large number of voluntary bodies that provide services as well. These may be charities specifically concerned with homelessness (such as Shelter and Crisis) but could include other organisations such the Salvation Army and local churches. The services that they provide vary greatly from area to area, but may include soup kitchens, hostels and day centres. Overall, provision of service to homeless people is patchy and often uncoordinated. Also presented are the difficulties encountered with multi-agency work including communication and the possibility of duplication of services.

Similar difficulties apply to the provision of mental health services to this population. The likely absence of a GP removes the most obvious first line of contact, and the lack of a fixed address will make it difficult to establish and maintain contact with an individual with regard to offering appointments, etc. As a result, these individuals are more likely to present when in a crisis and opportunities for dealing effectively with their illness at an earlier stage may be missed. As above, there is also likely to be difficulty in establishing which mental health team should take responsibility for these individuals because this is usually determined by address. As a result, homelessness is often deemed to be 'somebody else's problem' and the problems are not tackled head on.

Strategies for provision of mental health services

Clearly, the most important provision is that of access. Given the difficulties with access outlined above, the traditional means will work less well and so different approaches will be required. Resources need to be more directly available, and this could be accomplished (for example) by having community psychiatric nurses visit homeless shelters or hostels on a routine basis. They could also provide additional formal or informal training to hostel staff to help with early identification of mental illness.

The establishment of a specialist homeless team could also be of benefit. Such a team could direct its funding at recruiting and employing staff with appropriate skills, and would be able to build permanent links with charities and other organisations that already work with homeless people. It would be able to liaise with the community mental health teams so that transfer could be smoothly organised as people found accommodation and hence ceased to be homeless.

It will also be important, once cases have been identified, that a single person takes on responsibility for managing all aspects of his or her own care. The Care Programme Approach framework could be used, with the care coordinator taking on additional responsibilities for involving mental health, social services, housing, etc. Holding regular review meetings is also of value and helps in providing appropriate handover to conventional services. Good communication between the agencies involved and also with the patients themselves is clearly very important, and is of great importance in maintaining engagement.

Conclusion

Homeless people are a challenging group with complex needs in many areas, mental health being not least among them. The existing models of service are not well suited to serving them, and there is a need for new approaches. These must include increased integration and flexibility of care, with good integration of a range of services (including social work and housing, benefits, as well as mental health care).

There is a need for more research to be done into epidemiology, diagnosis and treatment of mental illness among homeless people, and for greater education of all involved in their care. The needs of homeless people are poorly met by existing services, and it is only by original thinking and willingness to be flexible that mental health services will be able to meet those needs adequately.

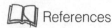 References

Scott J. Homelessness and mental illness. *British Journal of Psychiatry* 1993; 162: 314–324.

Tudor Hart J. The inverse care law. *Lancet* 1971; i: 405–412.

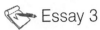 Essay 3

'Describe the challenges posed to mental health services by issues of ethnicity, and explain how the assessment and treatment of mental illness in these groups may differ from the general population.'

Introduction

Ethnic minorities in the UK can be simply defined as all those who do not consider themselves to fall within the 'white British' group. In the past, terms such as 'race' or 'culture' have been used or people have described themselves simply in terms of their appearance. However, these approaches are too narrow, and the now-accepted phrase 'ethnic minority' conveys a sense of cultural and social identity that goes beyond simple biological factors.

Ethnic minorities by definition differ from the general population, but this fact and its implications have not always been fully appreciated. Ethnic minorities have often been marginalised and socially excluded, leading to accusations of 'institutional racism' being levied against the workings of the state (including statutory bodies such as the police, Social Services and the NHS). These accusations have proved to be justified on a number of occasions. The Stephen Lawrence inquiry was critical of the police, and the NHS has been specifically included in the Race Relations Act of 2000.

Mental health services are clearly not exempt from these challenges. The aim of this essay is to consider in detail how ethnic minority populations differ in terms of their mental health, and to consider some the implications of these differences.

Differences between ethnic minorities and the general population

Clearly, an important question is whether and to what extent issues of mental health are different among ethnic minorities compared with the general population. The EMPIRIC study (Sproston and Nazroo, 2002) set out to investigate this; the overall finding was that there was no overall difference in rates of disease between different ethnic groups, but that it was very difficult to draw firm conclusions from these results. However, although there may be no overall difference in rates of disease, there are many other important differences to be considered in terms of illness, presentation, treatment and susceptibility to illness.

1. Different illnesses

Culture-bound syndromes are by definition mental illness presentations that occur only in certain ethnic minorities. They are often closely allied to cultural beliefs that might persist in a particular culture (eg the phenomenon of *dhat* is allied to a cultural belief concerning the value of semen). It must also be remembered that Western society can be said to have culture-bound syndromes of its own, and eating disorders such as anorexia nervosa have been viewed in this light.

2. Different presentation of illness

As a result of significant cultural differences, the presentation of the same illness may be quite different among ethnic minority groups. In some groups of people symptoms of depression and anxiety commonly present as somatisation, with patients complaining of a wide range of physical symptoms (aches and pains, etc.) rather than complaining of low mood. Cultural background is known to have an influence on the content of delusions. Finally, issues of language and communication may be a further barrier, obscuring the presentation of the illness and possibly the fact that illness is present at all.

The work of Cantor-Graae and Selten (2005) revealed higher rates of schizophrenia among first- and second-generation immigrants, even when all factors were controlled for. There is again no clear explanation for why this should be the case.

Finally, the attitude towards the health service and with regard to when it is appropriate to seek help may be quite different. Certain groups may wait for much longer before involving the health services, or may not even be aware of the help that is available.

3. Different treatments

Research that has been conducted into the management of ethnic minorities has suggested that they are admitted to psychiatric hospitals more often (and more often involving the Mental Health Act) and that higher doses of antipsychotics are used. No clear reason has emerged for why this should be so, and these findings have added to the fears of 'institutional racism'.

4. Greater susceptibility to illness

Although the EMPRIC study (Sproston and Nazroo, 2002) did not reveal any significant difference in rates of illness between populations, there are a number of reasons why those in ethnic minorities might be more prone to mental illness. The ever-present problem of racism may contribute to this, in terms of both racism in the population causing stress and anxiety and racism within the health service that may lead to misdiagnosis. Those who are first-generation immigrants will also have to contend with the impact of significant life events (moving to a new country, leaving friends and family behind, etc.).

Problems within the NHS

There have been a number of high-profile cases in which there have been failures within the NHS to take proper account of the needs of those in ethnic minorities. One of the best known of these resulted in the David 'Rocky' Bennett inquiry (Norfolk, Suffolk and Cambridgeshire Strategic Health Authority). David Bennett died after restraint while an inpatient at a medium secure unit. The findings of the report were that African–Caribbean people were over-represented among mental health inpatients, and were more likely to be subjected to coercion, regarded as dangerous and over-medicated. The report strongly recommended that NHS staff should receive training in cultural awareness and sensitivity.

The role of a specialist service

One possible way of addressing the difficulties listed above would be to establish separate, specialist services for treating ethnic minority groups. This is an approach that is gaining favour in some circles because it is felt to demonstrate clearly a commitment to avoiding discrimination, which is the legal duty of the NHS under the terms of the Race Relations Act. The advantages and disadvantages of such an approach have been debated in a number of public forums (eg Bhui and Sashidaran, 2003)

The case in favour of a specialist service is that the current inequalities (as described above) are unacceptable and that the current model of service provision is clearly not meeting needs sufficiently. Establishing specialist services for subgroups would allow the development of a specific skills base, which was suited to the needs of that population, and may also encourage engagement of these groups.

On the other hand, the evidence from the EMPIRIC study (Sproston and Nazroo, 2002) does suggest that the differences in actual illness rates are not as large as originally thought. The differences observed in outcome and management are a function of institutional factors within the health service. Establishing separate services would simply reinforce the impression of separation and isolation and increase stigma, and would not help with rooting out racism in the service. The other difficulties are logistical ones – how many different specialist services would be required, and how would the minority groups be defined? To run a separate service for every possible ethnic grouping would be impossible, so many of the difficulties will remain.

Conclusion

Developing services to meet the needs of ethnic minority populations in the UK is a challenging task. The emergence of evidence to suggest that underlying rates of illness differ little between populations has suggested that the observed differences in treatment and outcome result directly from the service itself. The charge of 'institutional racism' has been levelled at the NHS before, and at least to some degree has been found to be justified.

Some have suggested that specialist services for addressing the needs of these patients should be set up, but to do so would reinforce the isolation and separation of these groups. Instead, the whole of the NHS (mental health services included) should be educated and trained in dealing with people of all backgrounds, and racism should be ruthlessly rooted out. The findings of the EMPIRIC study (Sproston and Nazroo, 2002) need to be confirmed by further work, and also more evidence is required to establish how the needs of different populations vary in terms of assessment and treatment of their illnesses.

There is clearly much to be done, but addressing these issues will result in a health service that is non-discriminatory and acts in the best interests of all. The spectre of institutional racism can be buried once and for all.

References

Bhui K, Sashidaran SP. Should there be separate psychiatric services for ethnic minority groups? *British Journal of Psychiatry* 2003; 182: 10–12.

Cantor-Graae E, Selten J. Schizophrenia and migration – a meta-analysis and review. *American Journal of Psychiatry* 2005; 162: 12–24.

Norfolk, Suffolk and Cambridgeshire Strategic Health Authority. Independent inquiry into the death of David Bennett. December 2003.

Sproston K, Nazroo J (eds). *Ethnic Minority Psychiatric Illness Rates in the Community (EMPIRIC) – Quantitative report*. London: Department of Health, 2002.

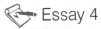 Essay 4

'Suicide cannot be prevented and to attempt to do so represents a waste of resources. Critically discuss this statement with reference to methods of risk assessment.'

Introduction

Suicide has been defined as 'a wilful self-inflicted life-threatening act resulting in death'. It is a relatively rare event, occurring in 11 in every 10 000 of the population per year. However, any suicide is associated with considerable distress for family and friends, which is fuelled by the notion that the death might have been prevented. However, this is no easy task and in many cases there has been no warning at all before the event that the individual was contemplating killing him- or herself. The National Confidential Enquiry into Suicide and Homicide reported that approximately 25% of people committing suicide have been in contact with mental health services in the previous year, and that 16% were psychiatric inpatients at the time of death.

However, the notion of preventability has fuelled Government policy, and the *Health of the Nation* document (Department of Health, 1998) aimed for a 15% reduction in the suicide rate overall by 2000, along with a general decrease in suicides among those with severe mental illness. These targets were achieved, but it is not clear to what extent this was the result of Government intervention. The National Service Framework for Mental Health (DH, 1999) promised a further decrease of 20% by 2010, and set out a variety of measures as part of Standard 7. These measures are predominately aimed at primary care, although they also include measures in prison populations.

There is clearly a significant political will to the effect that suicide can be prevented, and considerable resources have been directed towards accomplishing this (although the efficacy of these measures is unproven). It does, however, seem unduly negative to suggest that suicide cannot be prevented. The aim of this essay is to consider the arguments for and against the preventability of suicide, and to explore the effects of suicide prevention strategies.

In favour of preventability

There are many proponents of the view that suicide is preventable. First of all, the fact that rates have declined as described above after various Government initiatives is encouraging, although there is little evidence that this overall decline results directly from any particular intervention. However, there is no doubt that there are certain measures that can be shown to have a direct impact on suicide. These generally consist of reducing access to methods of suicide, and the most striking example is the sharply decreased rates of completed suicide after the switch from toxic coal gas to non-toxic natural gas in the 1970s. More recently, the total number of paracetamol tablets allowed to be sold at one time has been reduced, and co-proxamol (which contains dextropropoxyphene and paracetamol, the former being particularly dangerous in overdose) is to be withdrawn from the UK market altogether. There is now good evidence that reducing the size of paracetamol packs has had a significant impact on deaths from paracetamol overdoses (Hawton et al., 2004).

Second, an impact can be made on suicide indirectly by taking steps to improve the lot of those with mental health problems generally. Those with mental illness are still subject to stigma, and there have been attempts recently by the Royal College to educate the general public with a view to reducing this (such as the Changing Minds campaign). If the public can be educated and the negative attitudes corrected, those with a mental illness who might contemplate suicide may be more willing to seek help sooner and hence avert a crisis.

The Care Programme Approach (CPA) has formalised the ongoing follow-up of psychiatric patients. It is intended to be beneficial for all aspects of mental health, but it may have an impact on suicide as part of this. The designation of a named keyworker should promote continuity of care, and regular review meetings should reduce the chance of problems developing undetected. The additional support and structure provided by the CPA framework should allow the patient to feel better supported and provides a clear pathway for obtaining help.

As described above, reducing access to means is a proven method of decreasing suicide rates, although the published work often refers to a reduction in rates using that particular method rather than suicide rates in general. The reduction in rates of paracetamol overdose was followed by an increase in ibuprofen overdose, although the overall death rate did not change.

Given the relatively high percentage of deaths by suicide occurring in hospital inpatients, there is a clear mandate for further improving the safety of hospital wards. Measures should be taken to remove possible ligature points, install collapsing curtain rails and barricade-proof doors, ensure that patients can be observed if appropriate, and educate staff. The concept of the hospital as a place of safety needs to be robustly defended.

A new approach to managing self-harm and suicide is emerging in the form of psychological therapies. In particular, Linehan's dialectic behavioural therapy is thought to have specific impact on reducing acts of self-harm. This therapy has been derived from aspects of cognitive–behavioural therapy and is used among patients with borderline personality disorder and recurrent self-harm. However, it is possible that it could be used more broadly to address self-harm in patients with other diagnoses. There is a need for more research to be done to establish conclusively the use of such therapy.

There is much debate at present about the process of risk assessment. Historically, assessment of risk (of both self-harm and harm to others) has been carried out by psychiatrists, and other professionals, as part of the clinical interview. As a result the extent and quality of the risk assessment varies markedly between professionals. There has been much interest in so-called 'structured professional judgements' (Oyebode, 2005), such as the HCR-20, which provide a framework for considering risk. Although these are not without their problems, a standardised approach used across professions is likely to improve the standard of risk assessment overall and also allow for ease of comparison of risk across time.

Against preventability

It is important to remember, when considering preventability, that suicide is a rare event. The process of risk assessment should attempt to identify those who are likely to commit suicide, and so can be thought of in terms of a predictive test. The literature and terminology of such testing can hence be applied. The positive predictive value of a test for suicide will be low, given the rarity of it as an event. This means that the proportion of those with a positive test who go on to commit suicide will be low, limiting the usefulness of the test in practice. Similarly, any intervention aimed specifically at preventing suicide will have a very high number needed to treat. This means that a large number of people will need to be 'treated' (eg admitted to hospital or given intensive home treatment support) in order to prevent one suicide. This is likely to give rise to questions of cost-effectiveness when considering treatment based on the outcome of a test.

There are difficulties even in collecting information about suicide for the purpose of better risk assessment. Clearly, it is very difficult to get a clear idea about the patient's mental state after the suicide although efforts towards doing this have been made with the so-called 'psychological postmortems'. A further complication is that in some cases those dying by suicide did not actually intend to die, but rather to draw attention to themselves by an act of deliberate self-harm that went further than originally intended.

These difficulties are compounded by the fact that suicide is generally under-reported. A coroner's court can record a verdict of suicide only if there is sufficient evidence to show conclusively that this was the cause of the death. Often in cases where suicide is suspected there is insufficient evidence, and so an open verdict is recorded. As a result, studies of suicide must either keep to definite verdicts of suicide and risk excluding relevant data, or re-examine coroner's evidence, which may be very time-consuming and ultimately inconclusive.

Much attention is directed towards mental health services when discussing issues of suicide and its prevention, but it should be remembered that, according to the National Confidential Enquiry (Appleby et al., 2001), only 25% of suicides had been in contact with mental health services before death. Therefore, most suicides could not have been detected easily by mental health professionals in their daily work. It must therefore be concluded that many people who go on to commit suicide showed no signs that they were about to do so and had taken adequate steps to prevent suspicion or discovery. To prevent such events is clearly an extremely difficult, even impossible task.

Implications for resources

It is always a difficult task to make a judgement about whether it worth expending resources on a particular area. In terms of preventing suicide, it is clearly not possible to measure the number of suicides prevented, because one can never know whether an individual would have gone on to complete suicide if the preventive measures had not been in place.

Having considered the arguments above, it seems reasonable to conclude that, although there are significant difficulties in preventing suicide, there are certain groups that are at a much higher risk, so targeting measures at these populations is more likely to result in success. Also, many of the measures proposed as having an impact on suicide (such as reducing stigma and promoting public understanding and awareness of mental illness) are likely to have beneficial effects in other ways towards easing the problems associated with mental illness, and hence the overall burden on mental health services.

Conclusion

The preventability of suicide is a contentious area, and debate is likely to continue among psychiatrists and also within Government. Suicide remains an important but rare cause of death, although it is likely to retain a high profile given the emotive nature of any suicide. It is important that psychiatrists be involved in Government policy concerned with reducing suicides, because without informed professional input there is a risk of political solutions being introduced that are of questionable clinical validity. It needs to be made clear that risk assessments can under- or over-estimate the real risk, and that predicting the future in this way remains an inexact science.

The best chance of reducing suicide rates is to target high-risk groups with simple measures (such as reducing access to means), but this should not be to the exclusion of all others. Although psychiatrists have an important role to play, it should be remembered that in 75% of cases they would not have seen the individual concerned for at least 1 year, and the person would have been much more likely to have seen their GP or family members. As such, there is great need for education of all doctors and the general public. As with many aspects of mental illness, greater public awareness is vital if improvements are to be seen.

To return to the original statement, it is needlessly negative to say that resources directed at preventing suicide are wasted. It is, however, important to be pragmatic about the degree to which change can be effected and not to have unrealistic expectations. Suicide should not be singled out over other aspects of mental health, however, given its rarity compared with mental illness in general.

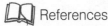 References

Appleby et al. *Safety First Report of the National Confidential Inquiry into Suicide and Homicide by People with Mental Illness*. London: The Stationery Office, 2001.

Department of Health. *The Health of the Nation – A Policy Assessed*. London: Department of Health, 1998.

Department of Health. *The National Service Framework for Mental Health*. London: Department of Health, 1999.

Hawton K et al. UK legislation on analgesic packs: before and after study of long term effect on poisionings. *British Medical Journal* 2004; 329: 1076–1079.

Oyebode F. Suicide, national enquiries and professional judgement. *Advances in Psychiatric Treatment* 2005; 11: 81–83.

General adult psychiatry

 Essay 1

'Mental health services have no role in the management of patients with personality disorders. Critically discuss this statement with reference to the evidence.'

Introduction

Personality disorders are defined in the ICD-10 as 'a severe disturbance in the characterological constitution and behavioural tendencies of the individual, usually involving several areas of personality and nearly always associated with considerable personal and social disruption'. These disturbances can take many forms, but perhaps the most difficult to deal with are the antisocial and emotionally unstable (borderline) types. As a result of the disruptions caused, these people regularly come into contact with psychiatrists and in some cases the criminal justice system, but it has often proved very difficult to find ways of producing a lasting improvement in their condition.

There has recently been increasing discussion and debate surrounding the validity of diagnosing personality disorder as a mental illness that requires treatment. The public profile has also been raised with the recent discussions about those with 'dangerous and severe personality disorders'. There are many conflicting views concerning who should be responsible for managing these people. Mental health services have traditionally played a major part, and to say that they have no role to play seems a very simplistic point of view.

The aim of this essay is briefly to review the classification and diagnosis of personality disorder, the relationship between personality disorder and mental illness, and the role of mental health services and other services in their management.

Classification and diagnosis of personality disorder

There have been many attempts to define personality disorders in general, one of which was given in the Introduction. An important feature is the enduring nature of the difficulties, which usually become clear around adolescence.

The many difficulties presented by personality disorder are mirrored by great difficulty in strictly defining and diagnosing them. The two main diagnostic schemes used in psychiatry (the ICD-10 and DSM-IV) differ slightly in their approach. The DSM-IV uses three 'clusters' to divide up the various subtypes, and uses slightly different terminology from the ICD-10 for some (eg ICD-10 has the 'emotionally unstable' category). In both schemes, the criteria tend to be rather vague. Attempts have been made to devise structured instruments for assessing personality such as Mann et al.'s (1981) 'Standardised Assessment of Personality', but these have not been universally adopted and none has attained 'gold standard' status.

Some have argued that categorical classification systems such as these are not suitable, and instead a dimensional classification system should be used. Again, some systems have been proposed and used in certain quarters, but none has gained universal acceptance.

Clearly, then, when discussing personality disorder, it is important to remember that patients with this diagnosis are a heterogeneous group.

Is a personality disorder a mental illness?

When considering whether mental health services should be involved, an important question is whether or not personality disorder can be considered to be a mental illness. There is a body of opinion that says that, rather than being a mental illness, personality disorder represents the extreme end of the normal spectrum of personality. The difficulty surrounding diagnosis described above is also a contributory factor – Lewis and Appleby (1988) found that the diagnosis was given to those whom doctors simply did not like. Certainly, classifying personality disorder is much more complex than with other mental illnesses, and this argues against it being considered alongside them.

However, there is considerable overlap between the difficulties of those with personality disorder and the difficulties of those with other well-recognised mental illnesses. Obsessive–compulsive (or anankastic) personality disorder is closely related to obsessive–compulsive disorder, and may simply be an extreme manifestation of it. Similarly, those with borderline personality disorder often demonstrate quasi-psychotic symptoms. There is also a considerable amount of co-morbidity (eg with depression) that must be considered. It appears logical that the expertise of psychiatrists in treating those with mental illness would be useful in treating similar problems presented by personality disorders.

Can personality disorders be treated?

Perhaps the most important question when considering the role of mental health services is whether personality disorders can be successfully treated. The main role of the psychiatrist in management of mental illness is to identify and implement appropriate treatment, and arguably if the disorder cannot be treated the role for the doctor is limited.

The treatment of personality disorder by drugs or psychological therapies is a subject in which there has been great interest. A recent review has summarised the body of literature on both of these interventions (Bateman and Tyrer, 2004a, 2004b). Personality disorder is currently being considered as at least potentially treatable, and possible avenues for treatment are being explored.

In terms of psychological therapies, the work is more advanced and there is more evidence available. There is a range of approaches that have been tried, including Ryle's cognitive analytic therapy, Linehan's dialectic behavioural therapy, Beck's cognitive–behavioural therapy and the therapeutic community 'milieu' approach. There remains no convincing evidence that favours any one of these over another, but there does seem to be some benefit from intervening rather than not.

Drug treatments are commonly used, and often those with personality disorders may be on several different classes and types of drugs. The rationale behind the choice of these drugs is often unclear, as is the benefit derived from them. However, recent work by Cloninger et al. (1993) has begun to suggest a neurobiological rationale for using drugs, in which different neurotransmitters are linked with different behaviour patterns (eg dopamine with novelty seeking). By analysing the pattern of behaviour and prescribing a drug with an appropriate action, improvements could be brought about. However, although this is an enticing model, there is as yet no conclusive clinical evidence to support these findings.

The role for other services

The final point to consider is who else might take responsibility for managing those with personality disorders if the mental health services do not. One point of view is that to give any treatment for personality disorder (whether psychological or pharmacological) is to medicalise the problems in a way that encourages the individuals not to take responsibility for their own actions ('it's not me, it's my illness'). The consequences of their actions may result in social disadvantage or deprivation (eg DSM-IV cluster C) or perhaps in criminal acts (eg DSM-IV cluster B). Social Services and the criminal justice system already have mechanisms in place for addressing such areas.

The criminal justice system has the ability to hold individuals to account for the consequences of their actions, and following this route rather than diversion to mental health services may prevent reinforcement of the view that the 'illness' is somehow responsible. The courts already have at their disposal the means for dealing with mental illness, and the court would be in a position to decide if medical reports were needed and if a hospital disposal was appropriate. There is no doubt that some (although a small minority) of those with personality disorder can be dangerous, and again the courts have greater powers at their disposal than the mental health services for managing this. The recent debate about dangerous and severe personality disorders highlighted this, and there are now specialist units at some UK prisons set up to deal with personality disorders.

Social Services are able to investigate and intervene in cases of social deprivation or disadvantage that might result in cases of personality disorder, and although mental health services might have a role to play in advising them it could be argued that Social Services could take the lead. Financial and housing issues are often big problems for these individuals, and prompt addressing of these would be of great benefit in managing their distress.

Conclusion

There is still considerable debate on the question of who should be involved in the management of those with a personality disorder. The diagnosis itself is one that is difficult to make and lacks a universally agreed description or diagnostic scheme. The diagnosis can be a subjective one, and doctors have been guilty of over-diagnosing it in patients who are difficult to manage.

There is also disagreement over whether personality disorder is a mental illness at all, or rather an extreme end of the normal range of human behaviour. However, there are many areas of overlap with mental illness and also significant co-morbidity with other mental illnesses. There is an emerging body of evidence that supports treatment in a number of modalities (both drug and psychological), although as yet nothing conclusive has emerged.

Mental health services, Social Services and the criminal justice system have all been cited as having a role to play, and a case can be argued for any of them to be the main contact point. However, to say that mental health services have no role to play is a very narrow view that does not take account of the available evidence or of current practice. Further research is needed into both diagnosis and treatment of personality disorders, and cooperation between the various services involved needs to be improved. Overall, however, mental health services are likely to play a continuing and vital role in the treatment of this important and challenging group.

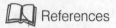 References

Bateman AW, Tyrer P. Psychological treatment for personality disorders. *Advances in Psychiatric Treatment* 2004a; 10: 378–388.

Bateman AW, Tyrer P. Drug treatment for personality disorders. *Advances in Psychiatric Treatment* 2004b; 10: 389–398.

Cloninger CR et al. A psychobiological model of temperament and character. *Archives of General Psychiatry* 1993; 50: 975–990.

Lewis G, Appleby L. Personality disorder: the patients psychiatrists dislike. *British Journal of Psychiatry* 1988; 153: 44–49.

Mann AH et al. The development and use of a standardised assessment of abnormal personality. *Psychological Medicine* 1981; 11: 839–847.

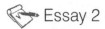 Essay 2

'Atypical antipsychotics in combination with modern community treatment spell the beginning of the end for inpatient care. Discuss this statement critically with reference to suitable evidence.'

Introduction

Schizophrenia is one of the most important of the illnesses seen and treated by psychiatrists. It is relatively common (with an incidence of 1%) and affects men and women equally. Approaches to diagnosis and treatment of schizophrenia have varied widely over the years, from the original kraepelinian view of 'dementia praecox' through to the modern idea of a chronic but manageable illness (much like diabetes mellitus in general medicine).

The advent of atypical antipsychotics has brought with it much hope with regard to the future treatment of schizophrenia, but these hopes have not always been fulfilled in clinical practice.

Although it might be tempting to imagine the end of inpatient treatment, it may be an unrealistic goal. The aim of this essay is to consider the early promise of atypical antipsychotics and their role in and impact on the treatment of schizophrenia. This will be applied to the provision of community services versus traditional hospital care.

Atypical antipsychotics

The coming of chlorpromazine in the 1950s heralded a new era in psychiatry, where previously unmanageable illness was found to respond to treatment. Expectations were high, and some even predicted the complete closure of all mental hospitals within 50 years. However, sustained use demonstrated numerous problems with this drug and others like it in terms of side effects (particularly extrapyramidal side effects and later tardive dyskinesia) and the emergence of treatment resistance.

The rise, fall and subsequent rebirth of clozapine, and in particular its use in treatment-resistant schizophrenia, brought with it renewed promise, and it is now considered to be the exemplar of the atypical antipsychotic. Over recent years, drug companies have directed considerable research efforts towards finding other drugs, all of which have in common a reduced propensity for extrapyramidal side effects, a different receptor-binding profile, a great deal of promise and (usually) a higher price. The reduction in side effects is said to increase tolerance and hence compliance with drugs, which should in turn lead to improved symptom control and so less need for inpatient stays.

On the face of it, the argument for using atypicals seems persuasive. However, despite the best efforts of the drug industry there is no absolutely conclusive evidence that atypicals are universally superior to their typical counterparts. First, with the possible exception of clozapine the currently available atypicals have not been used or studied to the same degree or over the same time period as the typicals. It remains possible that there are long-term effects of using these drugs of which we are as yet unaware. There has been recent controversy over the role of these drugs in the development of hyperglycaemia and diabetes mellitus, a chronic illness that carries with it a good deal of physical and psychological morbidity (eg Taylor, 2003).

Second, the evidence for the efficacy of the drugs themselves is generally little different for typicals and atypicals. The oft-quoted meta-analysis of Geddes et al. (2000) did not find a significant advantage for either group when compared with the other.

Third, there is a significant cost impact to be considered. Atypicals are much newer and many are still subject to patents. The drug companies are keen to recoup the substantial development costs, and this is reflected in the relatively high price of these products. Even clozapine, which is now quite old, is expensive because of the need for funding the patient-monitoring schemes. However, the recent arrival of other brands of clozapine should promote competition for business and a lowering of prices.

Are community models of care the best targets?

Resources in mental health as in the entire health service are limited, and careful consideration must be given to how they are used. The current model for psychiatric practice in the UK is primarily community based, and as cited in the title of the essay some would advocate that newer drugs and modern methods of practice pave the way for further expansion of community services.

There are a number of positive arguments for this point of view. History has taught the danger of the Goffman-esque 'Total Institution', and political pressure has led to the closure of the old asylums that were characteristic of such institutions. Admission to modern acute psychiatric hospitals can be very difficult for patients and their families, and safely maintaining people in their home environment should be more conducive to promoting recovery. It also helps to lessen some of the stigma attached to mental illness in general and schizophrenia in particular.

With regard to the role of atypicals, it is argued that, because these drugs are better tolerated and cause fewer side effects, many of the precipitating factors for admission to hospital (poor compliance, forced change of medication, etc.) have been diminished, if not removed altogether.

However, there are also a number of counter-arguments. The first is that atypical antipsychotics do not work effectively for every patient. The tolerability is not always as good as hoped for, and there are many other reasons for non-compliance seen in these populations besides tolerability (eg insight, patient preference). Second, many would argue that there will always be a role for hospital inpatient care, and neglecting it in favour of further investment in community services is storing up trouble for the future. There is much in the hospital that cannot easily be done in the community, and at times removal from home is necessary to avoid further pressure on mental state. The concentration of medical and nursing staff with rapid access to consultant opinion is often more difficult to achieve in the community. Third, drug treatment has no effect on incidence of disease, and there is no evidence that incidence is changing. Modern initiatives such as early intervention teams are trying to address this problem, but the evidence base is not robust and it is too early to make judgements about how successful they have been. This, accompanied by a high level of ignorance among the general public (despite the best efforts of the College such as the 'Changing Minds' campaigns), means that the first episode of psychosis may often go unrecognised until a crisis point is reached, often requiring rapid admission to hospital (sometimes requiring the Mental Health Act). The concept of the hospital as a 'place of safety' is a crucial one that cannot be easily be replaced by community teams.

Conclusion

Atypical antipsychotics have many benefits, and they are a useful and valuable addition to the psychiatrist's arsenal of drugs. However, they are a not a panacea and have their own flaws, many of which relate to our relative inexperience in their use and ignorance of long-term side effects. Although aspects of their use should mean that hospital admission may be needed less frequently, it remains an essential part of psychiatric care. To divert resources away would be short sighted, and what is required is a strong community network of well-trained professionals backed up by a robust and well-resourced hospital for times when it will inevitably be needed.

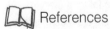 References

Taylor D. Antipsychotic prescribing – time to review practice. *Psychiatric Bulletin* 2002; 26: 401–402.

Geddes JR et al. Atypical antipsychotics in the treatment of schizophrenia – systematic overview and meta-regression analysis. *British Medical Journal* 2000; 321: 1371–1376.

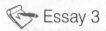 Essay 3

'Bipolar affective disorder should be treated only with lithium. Discuss this statement critically with reference to appropriate evidence.'

Introduction

Bipolar affective disorder is defined in the ICD-10 as 'A disorder characterised by repeated episodes in which the patient's mood and activity levels are significantly disturbed'. These episodes may be manic in which there is elevated mood with increased energy and activity, or depressive in which the opposite occurs. It is a serious and important mental illness that can have a devastating impact on the lives of its sufferers and their friends and family.

Traditionally, lithium has been the mainstay of treatment, and historically few would have disagreed with this statement that only lithium should be used. However, in recent years opinion has begun to change and there are a now a range of available treatments, although the evidence for these is variable in quantity and quality. It should also be remembered that treatment for bipolar disorder (as with treatment in general) consists not only of drugs but also of psychological and social interventions.

The aim of this essay is to consider the case for treatment, and discuss which treatments are available in all modalities. In conclusion, a judgement shall be made about whether lithium is indeed the only treatment that should be used.

The case for treatment

When discussing treatment for any illness, it is important to establish why the illness should be treated and what the consequences might be if left inadequately treated or not treated at all.

The DSM-IV includes for many of its entries a consideration about the impact of the illness on social and occupational functioning, and there is little doubt that bipolar affective disorder can have a significant impact on both. It tends to follow a more chronic and relapsing course than unipolar depression, and sufferers are much more likely to attempt suicide than those with other diagnoses (Dilsaver et al., 1994). There is a considerable potential for risk, in terms of both suicide and self-harm when depressed, or the consequences of mania (promiscuity, spending money, etc.). Compliance with treatment may also be more an issue because being hypomanic or manic can be ego-syntonic.

These issues together make a good case for the treatment of bipolar affective disorder including using the Mental Health Act should it prove necessary. Treatment, as always, should be considered in terms of biological, psychological and social interventions.

Biological interventions

Drug treatment for bipolar affective disorder can itself be further categorised into acute treatment and prophylaxis of mania.

Traditionally, lithium has been the mainstay of treatment for both in the UK. Lithium salts were originally found to be effective by Cade in the late 1940s, and since then have been much researched. There is no doubt that it is effective, but there are a number of well-known difficulties associated with its use. It has a narrow therapeutic window that can make dosing difficult, and it is often poorly tolerated because of unpleasant side effects. There is a wide range of interactions with other drugs, and regular monitoring of serum levels is needed. There is always a potential risk of lithium toxicity which can be life threatening. Relapse rates after stopping lithium have been reported to be as high as 50%, and rebound mania on discontinuation is well known. It is also becoming increasingly clear that it is less useful for rapid cycling mania, affective psychosis and bipolar depression.

Practice in the USA has historically tended towards the use of antipsychotics in the acute phase, although lithium is used for maintenance as a result of other difficulties associated with long-term antipsychotic use (such as tardive dyskinesia). With the advent of the atypical antipsychotics interest in using them as anti-manic agents has revived, and olanzapine now has a licence for acute mania in the UK. It has also been suggested that atypical antipsychotics may be useful for prophylaxis of mania, and it is hoped that there will be fewer problems with side effects from long-term use.

Anticonvulsant medications are also being used for acute mania because they have been found to have mood-stabilising properties. In particular, semisodium valproate (marketed as Depakote) and carbamazepine have been given a licence for this use. They are gradually becoming more popular, and there is an increasing body of evidence to support their use. The use of anticonvulsants for prophylaxis is established in the USA where sodium valproate is used. In the UK, carbamazepine has a licence for prophylaxis and lamotrigine is also used off-label.

A Cochrane review in 2001 (Burgess et al., 2001) in the UK considered the available evidence, and eventually concluded that lithium should be used as the first choice. However, this was based more on the fact that evidence for other drugs was insufficient rather than that lithium was proved better. The BALANCE study, which will compare lithium with valproate and a combination of the two, is ongoing and the results are eagerly awaited.

Psychological treatments

The use of psychological interventions such as cognitive–behavioural therapy in unipolar depression is well established, and the recent NICE guidelines recommend their use. They also have much to offer sufferers of bipolar disorder. First of all, work on identifying prodromal signs and relapse signatures can be very helpful in predicting relapse, and such simple measures can allow the patient to identify signs of relapse early and seek appropriate help before a crisis is reached.

Cognitive therapy has a role as well, as demonstrated in a recent randomised controlled trial by Lam et al. (2003). This work compared cognitive therapy plus medication with medication alone, and found that the intervention group has significantly fewer episodes. These episodes were also shorter and resulted in fewer admissions, and the patients were more compliant with medication.

Simple measures such as psychoeducation can also have a significant impact. It is well known that life events (Brown and Harris, 1978) of all kinds can precipitate relapse, so advice to that effect will allow sufferers to take extra care during predictable life events (such as moving house or getting married) and seek help promptly after unpredictable ones (death of a loved one, etc.). Circadian rhythm disruption is associated with relapse, and so general lifestyle advice about the importance of regular and sufficient sleep can be given. There are clearly other lifestyle factors (such as choice of occupation) that are relevant, and the implications of these should also be discussed.

Social interventions

Social interventions that are likely to be beneficial are common to many mental illnesses. Simple measures such as adequate housing, financial provision and community support are all likely to improve prognosis if they are correctly dealt with. Social workers have an important role to play in all three of these areas; they can assist in identifying suitable placements, dealing with benefit applications and arranging community involvement through day centres, work programmes, etc. Finding employment can be difficult (not least because of the stigma attached to mental illness) and so assistance with finding a sympathetic employer is also likely to be of great value.

The importance of addressing social factors should not be underestimated, and many factors associated with relapse can be precipitated by undesirable social factors, eg living in unsuitable housing may result in difficulties sleeping, and socially isolated individuals may find it difficult to find help except in a crisis.

Conclusion

Bipolar affective disorder is an important mental illness, and there are a variety of treatment strategies available in all modalities. There are a number of drug treatments including lithium salts, anticonvulsants and antipsychotics, although the evidence base for the latter two groups is incomplete. There are good reasons to prefer some of these agents over lithium in many individuals, especially if there have been previous difficulties with lithium or where other factors are at play (eg the patient is taking medication that may interact with lithium). There is also a range of other non-drug treatments that are helpful in combination or alone, and simple social measures must not be neglected.

Lithium is by no means the only treatment available for bipolar affective disorder, and to say that it alone should be used is an exceedingly narrow statement. It does remain a viable option and an important drug, and it still deserves its place in the psychiatrist armoury. However, alternatives should be considered and where possible the patient should be involved in decision-making. Continued scientific investigation into all the available treatments is required to establish their efficacy, and further work aimed at discovering new treatments would also be valuable. Such evidence will inform prescribing decisions and ensure that patients receive the best and most suitable treatment for a serious and potentially devastating illness.

References

Brown GW, Harris TO (eds). *Social Origins of Depression: A study of psychiatric disorder in women.* London: Tavistock, 1978.

Burgess et al. Lithium for maintenance treatment of mood disorders. *The Cochrane Database of Systematic Reviews.* Issue 3 Art. No. CD003013, 2001.

Cade JF. Lithium salts in the treatment of psychotic excitement. *Medical Journal of Australia* 1949; 2: 349–352.

Dilsaver SC et al. Suicidality in patients with pure and depressive mania. *American Journal of Psychiatry* 1994; 151: 1312–1315.

Lam DH et al. A randomized controlled study of cognitive therapy for relapse prevention for bipolar affective disorder: outcome of the first year. *Archives of General Psychiatry* 2003; 60: 145–152.

Old age psychiatry

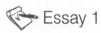 Essay 1

'The increase in life expectancy is one of the biggest challenges facing society. Discuss this phrase with particular reference to the care of those with dementia.'

Introduction

Life expectancy can be defined as the number of years that an individual is expected to live, as derived from population statistics. There is no doubt that life expectancy in the UK is increasing. Over the past 20 years, it has become increasingly apparent that people are living longer and enjoying prolonged good health. There are a number of reasons for this, not least the improved quality of health care and improved access to it. The impact of the introduction of the National Health Service and the 'free at point of use' principle is still being felt, and this is reflected in increased life expectancy. Living conditions, nutrition and good promotion of a healthy lifestyle have also contributed.

Clearly, this change in the demographic structure has profound implications for society. Many have noted with alarm the 'inverted pyramid' that is developing in which there are many more older than younger people. This has an obvious financial implication (fewer tax payers and more drawing pensions), but also a significant impact on health services and families in society.

This essay aims to discuss the major implications for health services and carers, and go on to consider in more detail the impact upon those who care for sufferers of dementia.

Impact on health services

An ageing population brings with it many challenges to health services in general, and mental health services in particular. The needs of an ageing population may differ significantly from those of the younger adults. Chronic disease management becomes much more important, and the need for ongoing involvement and health promotion is increased. As people live for longer, they become more prone to 'wear-and-tear' illnesses such as osteoarthritis, and this brings with it the need for other services (such as occupational therapy and physiotherapy).

In terms of mental health, the most obvious illness of old age is that of dementia. Increased life expectancy clearly implies that patients with dementia will need to be managed for longer. There is also the risk of co-morbidity (both physical and mental illesses) that will need to be addressed. However, besides this there will be more cases of other mental illness in old age such as depression and late-onset or very-late-onset schizophrenia.

There has been debate for some time about how these challenges should be addressed by mental health services. The establishment of old age psychiatry as a separate speciality in 1988 recognised that a different approach was required. Debate has raged ever since over whether totally separate, specialist services were an advantage over an integrated approach involving all professionals.

The proponents of a specialist service argue that they provide a service tailored to the needs of elderly people, with great awareness of (for example) physical health needs. They are also able to involve specialist occupational therapy and physiotherapy in order to provide specific input. Old age services are also able to gain specialist knowledge in identifying and managing the presentation of mental illness in old age, which may differ significantly from the adult population.

The opponents claim that to separate people simply on the basis of their age is a needlessly reductionist strategy and can lead to numerous problems. First, it might be said to encourage ageist stereotypes and discourage those in general services from learning about how best to adjust their care to differing needs. Second, there is the risk of the discontinuity of care that may arise if a patient is unceremoniously 'handed over' once he or she reaches a certain age. Finally, there is often concern that well-researched specialist services may attract capable staff away from overstretched general services where they are needed most.

Impact on carers

Carers can be defined as those involved in looking after people with needs that they are unable to meet fully themselves. Usually, when discussing carers the term is taken to refer to those who care for people informally (ie they are not paid to do so professionally). Carers can be family or friends, and the role often begins as a small undertaking but gets more and more difficult as the patient's needs increase.

The immediate impact of increasing life expectancy is that of the increasing need for carers. More people living for longer will necessarily increase the numbers of those with chronic illnesses who require care. In terms of mental health, dementia again is the illness in which carers are most relevant.

Caring for someone with dementia can be difficult and challenging, although also rewarding. A significant percentage of carers find the work rewarding, although the stress imposed on them is very difficult to deal with. Until now, carers and their needs have often been ignored. They are often said to be the 'hidden patients' of our services. It has been estimated that the care provided by informal carers saves the NHS a considerable sum of money annually. This is only likely to increase as the population ages and more people require care. The consequences of continuing to ignore the needs of carers are great, in terms of both resources and the psychological morbidity of the carers themselves.

Oyebode has studied what underlies stress in carers. One of the main findings was that the behaviour of the patient, rather than the severity of the illness, was a predictor of stress. In terms of a patient with dementia, behavioural problems often form a significant component of the clinical presentation, so they are perhaps more likely than the carer of someone with a chronic physical illness suffering stress as a result of the caring role.

Supporting and providing information to carers

With the increasing recognition of the role of carers there has been a great deal of interest from Government and also from the Royal College of Psychiatrists in providing appropriate support to carers. The National Service Framework for Mental Health (Department of Health, 1999) specifically includes carers in Standard 6, saying that they should be involved in review processes and given a written care plan. This was echoed in the NSF for Older Adults (DH, 2001), which also included the needs of carers in the Standards set.

Legislation aimed at carers has also been introduced, although this has not always been successful. The Carers (Services and Provisions) Act of 1995 gave carers the right to request an assessment of needs from Social Services, but it did not place any obligation on Social Services to provide any specific assistance. However, this has been interpreted as a statement of intent to help, and has been successful in raising the profile of carers.

Practical resources for giving support should not be overlooked, because these can make a big difference. Carers often feel undervalued and ignored, and even simple measures can have great impact. The provision of short-term respite care can be a great help, even if it is only for a short space of time. The involvement of occupational therapy and physiotherapy can also be invaluable to aid with the practicalities of managing a needy patient. Patients with dementia often benefit from specialist occupational therapy provision such as life-story work.

Regular review, as provided for by the Care Programme Approach (CPA) framework, can also be of great help to carers, because it provides an opportunity for their voice to be heard and for concerns to be raised. Access to services is an important part of the NSF for Mental Health, and prompt response to changes in the patient's condition and the institution of appropriate intervention can help to avoid situations that impose the most stress on the carer.

Finally, the provision of appropriate information to carers so that they feel empowered and equipped is of great importance. There are a number of ways in which this might be accomplished. First, the Royal College of Psychiatrists has established the 'Partners in Care' scheme in association with the Princess Royal Trust for Carers. This scheme set out to raise the profile of carers and to provide resources for them. There is a variety of written material available that could be distributed by hospital outpatient departments or by community teams. It is also available on the internet, which is increasingly accessible. Patient support groups often closely involve carers, and these can provide a very useful resource when meeting others in similar circumstances.

It is also important that carers are well informed about the nature of the illness. In dementia, it is important that they are well informed about the likely course and prognosis, so that they have realistic expectations and also so that they can look out for unexpected changes and alert staff to them. Carers should be told about what help and support are available and how it can be accessed (especially out of hours, as stipulated in Standard 3 of the NSF for Mental Health). Overall, carers should be well informed and involved in the management of the patient, and should have access to support appropriate for their needs. This may range from simple support and advice to organising respite placement on an occasional or regular basis. Lastly, they should be aware of the importance of looking after their own health.

Conclusion

The ageing population in the UK presents very many challenges to society in general, and to mental health services in particular. The provision of services will have to adapt to these needs, and different solutions to the new problems presented will need to be found. The importance of carers is becoming increasingly recognised and effort by both the Government and the Royal College are to be welcomed. However, much more is needed and in particular legislation that compels greater assistance from Social Services. More research is required on the impact on services and also on the effectiveness of measures already employed on reducing the burden on carers.

These challenges will be with us for a long time to come, and it is only by developing effective services, backed by appropriate legislation, that progress will be made in this important area.

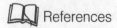 References

Department of Health. *The National Service Framework for Mental Health*. London: Department of Health, 1999.

Department of Health. *The National Service Framework for Older Adults*. London: Department of Health, 2001.

Oyebode J. Assessment of carers' psychological needs. *Advances in Psychiatric Treatment* 2003; **9**: 45–53.

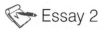 Essay 2

'Describe how the needs of older adults differ from the general population, and outline the arguments for and against the provision of specialist mental health services in this area.'

Introduction

Older adults may be defined as those over the age of 65, and they constitute an increasingly large section of the population. The population in the UK is ageing and life expectancy is increasing, so this group is set to increase still further. There are numerous challenges to health services posed by older adults, because their health care needs are in many ways different and more complex than those of younger people.

Mental health problems in older adults are similarly challenging. There is considerable psychiatric morbidity among older adults, both in terms of mental illnesses such as depression and schizophrenia and with regard to chronic conditions more common in old age such as dementia. The prevalence of depression in old age in 13.5% (Beekman et al., 1999), and older adults are more likely to be subject to life events such as the loss of a close relative, moving house. The prevalence of dementia also increases greatly as age increases – 2% at age 65, 10% at age 80 and 30% at age 90.

The establishment of mental health services for older adults is a relatively new development. The closure of the large mental hospitals resulted in the discharge of many long-stay patients. They were subsequently dispersed into the community, and the different needs of the old age population have subsequently emerged. Old age psychiatry was created as a speciality in 1988, and this formalised the recognition that the needs of this population were different. Older adults were specifically excluded from the National Service Framework for Mental Health (Department of Health, 1999), and instead their mental health needs were addressed in the NSF for Older Adults in 2001.

Wherever specialist services exist there is always debate about the justification for them, and old age is no different. The aim of this essay is to consider the case for and against the provision of a specialist service, the difficulties surrounding 'graduates' (ie those with long-standing illness who reach the 'cut-off' age of 65), and finally the arguments surrounding the treatability of dementia.

Older adults with mental health problems

Broadly speaking, older adults with mental health problems can be considered as belonging to two groups: 'graduates' and those experiencing their first episode of mental illness in later life.

Graduates are those with long-standing mental illness who are (or have been) in contact with general services and who reach the age of 65. They have often been on medication for a long time, and are more likely to be taking traditional 'typical' antipsychotics. They are also likely to be suffering from the well-documented side effects of these including movement disorders or extrapyramidal side effects. As a result of having suffered from mental illness for a long time, they are often socially isolated and may be alienated from families and sources of support. They may also have relatively poor physical health as a result of neglect or non-compliance with treatment or doctors' appointments.

Those suffering their first episode of mental illness in later life are quite different from the 'graduates'. The possibility of a physical cause for their presenting symptoms is much higher and needs to be rapidly excluded. There is increasing evidence to suggest that certain psychiatric symptoms may be the prodrome of a physical illness. One such example is Parkinson's disease; patients with this may often present initially with symptoms of depression before the movement disorder has become apparent. It may be that the effects on the dopamine system may exhibit themselves as mood symptoms before they are severe enough to affect movement. Similarly, 'vascular depression', in which subclinical ischaemic events produce symptoms of depression, has been described and may be a predictor of further vascular problems for the future.

Depression in old age has been studied in detail and found to be more likely to follow a chronic course and have a higher relapse rate than in the general population. Coupled with this is that fact that older adults are more likely to be exposed to life events (particularly 'exit' events such as the loss of a spouse, the need to move house).

The argument concerning a specialist service

There is no doubt that in many ways the needs of the older adult population are different from those of younger adults. Some would argue that this makes the case for separate, specialist services, but others argue that this is a false distinction and that general services should indeed be general in their approach.

In favour of a specialist service

A specialist skills base is needed when dealing with older adults, and many of these skills are not applicable in general services. The process of assessment needs to include mental, social and physical factors, but the problems identified and interventions required may be different.

The presentation of physical illness with psychiatric symptoms (eg thyroid problems, electrolyte imbalances, sensory deprivation such as deafness) is much more common in old age, and it is very important that this is recognised. Greater attention must be paid to reversible physical causes of such symptoms that might otherwise be needed in general adult populations. A specialist team will be able to establish links with medical teams at general hospitals and promote communication and exchange of information between the two. It is far more likely that older adults will be in contact with both general and psychiatric hospitals, and the smaller scale of a specialist service will make such links more practical to forge and maintain.

Domiciliary visits are a much greater part of old age psychiatry, often because associated issues such as mobility and physical illness may prevent attendance at outpatients, etc. Domiciliary visits require more time and effort than outpatient clinics, so a specialist service will take this load off the general services while at the same time being able to tailor its own provision accordingly. Day hospitals are again a service that is much more important in old age, and the running of these can be taken on by a specialist service and hence provide continuity of care. Finally, a specialist team will have the opportunity to forge close links with local residential or nursing homes, in which many of the patients seen will ultimately require placement.

It is also important to consider the needs of older adults in inpatient settings. General adult wards are often inappropriate for older adults because their needs are different. They are less likely to be admitted in a crisis, and the increased physical health needs require specific knowledge on the part of the doctors and nurses. Some old age psychiatry wards employ general nurses, or nurses with extensive general as well as mental health experience, for this reason. It would be difficult to justify such measures on a general acute psychiatric ward.

The increasing role for psychological interventions in the treatment of older adults with mental health problems also demands therapists skilled in such interventions, and administering the therapy may require a different approach from that used for younger adults. Also, there is some role for psychological therapies in dementia that would again require specific training. Such specialised roles would be more likely to flourish in a separate service where they could be utilised to the full.

Against a specialist service

Those opposed to a separate service advocate that the splitting up of the patient group into ever smaller chunks is ultimately detrimental to patient care and an inefficient use of resources. They point out that the result is a significant degree of duplication of services and there are more opportunities for breakdown in communication and for people to be overlooked in the transition from one to another.

First of all, the age cut-off of 65 is very arbitrary. The current needs and mental state of all patients aged 65 is likely to be very variable, so to say that all those aged 65 and older are better served by a separate service seems a strange judgement. It might be more appropriate to establish cut-offs based on level of functioning or disease course and progression, but generally (as in the NSF for Older Adults) age is used to define the two populations. This may lead to an abrupt termination of the relationship with the adult services once this age is reached, which patients may find very difficult to understand and which may even provoke relapse.

Second, connected with this is the argument that even within the population of over-65s the needs are very variable. It seems likely that the needs of the average 66 year old are likely to be very different from those of the average 86 year old, and yet they all fall under the same 'older adult' bracket. The logical extension of this is that there should be a 'younger older adult' service, which is clearly a ridiculous proposition. The opponents of separate services argue that all such divisions are therefore false, and one general service should adapt to the differing needs across the lifetime of the patient.

Third, the establishment of specialist services (often with considerable publicity and investment of resources) runs the risk of hastening the decline of the general services. Already in general medicine and surgery the dangers of super-specialisation have been seen, in which every doctor is capable of working only in a very narrowly defined area and relies on equally specialist colleagues for support in anything else. Even general practitioners have not been immune from specialisation! New, well-resourced services will tend to be attractive to capable staff because they are likely to be better resourced and provide better career opportunities. The result is de-skilling of the general services, which are left with less able staff in areas where good quality staff are most needed (this is akin to Tudor Hart's [1971] 'inverse care law').

Conclusion

The need for a different approach to managing older adults with mental health problems has been well established, and it is developing to meet the challenges posed. There are arguments on both sides about the value of specialist services, but policy is such that specialist services for older adults have been established almost universally. It is therefore of great importance that the services work together to ensure clear guidelines for transfer from one to the other and that the process of transition is managed well to avoid an abrupt cut-off.

The problem of graduates persists, and practice differs from place to place. The Royal College has recommended that, at the very least, all graduates should be identified and given a full multidisciplinary review to establish which service will best meet their needs. The Care Programme Approach is also important in formalising the process of follow-up and review.

The NSF for Older Adults has been helpful, but its inclusion of all aspects of health care has led to less emphasis being placed on mental health. National guidelines for running specialist services and improved resourcing of general services would be of value in ensuring good service provision for patients, irrespective of their age.

References

Beekman AT et al. Review of community prevalence of depression in later life. *British Journal of Psychiatry* 1999; 174: 307–311.

Department of Health. *The National Service Framework for Mental Health*. London: Department of Health, 1999.

Department of Health. *The National Service Framework for Older Adults*. London: Department of Health, 2001.

Tudor Hart J. The inverse care law. *Lancet* 1971; i: 405–412.

Forensic psychiatry

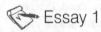 Essay 1

'The legacy of psychiatry in the early twenty-first century will be that it was the era in which hospitals were closed and prisons expanded. Discuss this statement with reference to the literature on forensic mental health services.'

Introduction

The face of psychiatry has changed dramatically over the past 20 years. The old system of predominately institutional care has been swept away and replaced with a community-based model. The role of the hospital and the role of the psychiatrist have also changed, and the implications of these changes are still emerging. These organisational changes have in turn led to changes in the way mental illness is managed, with more emphasis on treatment in the community. There have also been developments in new models of care, such as assertive outreach, early intervention.

However, at the same time some alarming trends have been noted in the criminal justice system. The prison population has been expanding rapidly to the point that many prisons are overcrowded and having difficulty in coping with the demands placed on them. Clearly, a need remains to manage challenging and dangerous behaviour, and there is considerable debate over whose role this actually is.

It has been suggested that the rapid increase in the prison population is directly linked to the de-institutionalisation of mental health, and that there is a group of individuals for whom institutional care of some form is inevitable. However, to reduce this to the statement in the question appears to be a gross oversimplification of the current situation. The aim of this essay is to consider the validity of the statement with reference to historical factors and the links between mental illness and offending behaviour.

History

Until the discovery of chlorpromazine in the 1950s, mental health care was defined by the confinement of the mad. Initially an informal process (often managed within families or small social groupings) it became formalised in Victorian times with the establishment of large asylums. These grew at great speed, and rapidly became notorious for poor living conditions and abuse of patients. However, no viable alternative was available and the asylums continued to grow.

The advent of viable treatment for mental illness with the increased refinement of pharmacological therapies began the process of decline. Political pressure was brought increasingly to bear, and the development of community-based models for the treatment of mental illness led to widespread closure of the asylums and dispersal of the patients to the communities from which they had for so long been excluded. By now, there are few of the old hospitals left and very often the buildings themselves have been disposed off. The community model is well established, and the hospital as a place of long-term stay no longer exists.

Expansion of the prison system

At the same time as this large-scale reduction of the numbers of patients in mental hospitals, the prison system has been undergoing dramatic expansion. Prison occupancy has increased by 50% in the past 10 years (Birmingham, 2004), and the prison service is having difficulty in coping with the great demands placed on it. Prisoners are subject to many of the problems that were encountered historically in the asylums, and it is known that they are vulnerable to developing mental health problems.

Fazel et al. (2002) reported that one in seven prisoners has a psychotic illness or major depression, and an Office of National Statistics survey (Singleton et al., 1998) revealed high rates of all mental illnesses in prisoners (with remand prisoners worse than sentenced prisoners).

It is not a simple matter to separate cause from effect – does being a prisoner place one at a higher risk of mental illness, or are those with mental illness at a higher risk of being imprisoned? This leads on to the question of whether there is a link between the end of institutional care (and hence the containment of many people with mental illness) and the subsequent surge in the prison population (which has been described as 'transinstitutionalisation' by Snowdon et al., 2002).

Mental illness and imprisonment

The question about whether the prison population has increased as a result of the closure of mental hospitals is not one that can be easily answered. The only way that this could be definitively answered would be if comprehensive data had been collected on the nature and composition of prison and hospital populations before and after the closure of the asylums (Reed, 2002). These data are not available, and would be very difficult to analyse if they were. It seems unlikely that there is a simple association between the two events. Prisoners with mental illnesses are not new, and reading accounts of prisons dating back over hundreds of years reveals records of 'demented' prisoners. Having said that, the lack of readily available hospital beds and the increasing difficulty in gaining admission to psychiatric hospitals may have had some effect on the number of people who cannot function in the community and as a result become entangled in the criminal justice system.

There are a number of reasons why those who have a mental illness may be more likely to be found in prison. First, they are more likely to be arrested, and after a court appearance are more likely to be remanded in custody than those without mental illness. Modern evidence also suggests that there is a slightly increased risk of violence among those with mental illness. Certain factors associated with mental illness (including homelessness, substance misuse and low social class) are also linked with offending behaviour and subsequent imprisonment, and also other aspects of mental illness (such as impulsivity in affective states or lack of planning or forethought) may make detection of offending behaviour more likely. Once in prison, mental illness (either pre-existing or arising anew) may not be detected or treated as rapidly as in the community (Birmingham et al., 1998). Mental illness is often missed at reception health screening, and prison officers are generally not sufficiently trained or skilled to detect such illness in existing prisoners, which may be masked by good behaviour.

One difficulty with the community model of mental health care is that it usually does not account for those who pass out of the community, whether to another location or to an environment such as a prison. 'Inreach' services and follow-up in prisons are rare, and court diversion or schemes of diversion at point of arrest are not universally implemented. As a result, patients may now end up being sent to prison when a hospital admission would be a more appropriate disposal. Although they may come into contact with forensic mental health services thereafter, the shortage of secure beds may make hospital treatment even more difficult to access. After leaving prison, even though their needs may not have changed the fact that they have a forensic 'career' may cause general services to be reluctant to take them back onto their caseload.

Conclusion

It is clearly an oversimplification to attribute the expansion of the prison population to the closure of the asylums. It is also impossible to support such an assertion without having access to detailed data on the populations that are not readily available. However, discussing the issue does raise a number of important points about the problems of mental illness in prisons and the role of the community mental health teams in dealing with such patients.

Forensic mental health services are expanding to take account of the expanding prisons, but at present demand outstrips supply. Mental disorder in prison is a significant problem and expanded services, along with further training of prison officers, are essential if it is to be addressed.

The community mental health model on the whole takes little account of those involved in the justice system, and frequently has little interface with it. The development and implementation of carefully constructed protocols for liaison between general and forensic services is clearly very important. Court diversion schemes are arrangements with local police that can be helpful in avoiding inappropriate admissions to prison.

The prisons are the last of the institutions to remain, and it is to be hoped that the legacy of community psychiatry will be closely allied to the recognition of the extent of mental illness in prisons and its effective management.

References

Birmingham L. Mental disorder and prisons. *Psychiatric Bulletin* 2004; 28: 393–397.

Birmingham L et al. A follow-up study of mentally disordered men remanded to prison. *Criminal Behaviour and Mental Health* 1998; 8: 202–213.

Fazel S et al. Serious mental disorders in 23000 prisoners: a systematic review of 62 surveys. *Lancet* 2002; 359: 545–550.

Reed J. Delivering psychiatric care to prisoners: problems and solutions. *Advances in Psychiatric Treatment* 2002; 8: 117–125.

Singleton et al. *Psychiatric Morbidity Among Prisoners in England and Wales*. London: Office of National Statistics, 1998.

Snowdon et al. Old age psychiatry services. *Psychiatric Bulletin* 2002; 26: 24–26.

Child psychiatry

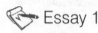 Essay 1

'How does the presentation, assessment and treatment of depression differ in children and adolescents compared with adults? Discuss the implications of the difference.'

Introduction

Depression is a common mental illness that is frequently encountered by psychiatrists. According to the report of US Surgeon General (1999), the prevalence of a depressive episode in the adult population is 6.5%, and other work has put the lifetime prevalence at 16% (psychiatric morbidity among adults living in a private household study). The impact of depression can be significant and it can cause impairments in social and occupational functioning.

Depression is seen in people of all ages, and so is of interest to child psychiatrists. It is particularly important to recognise depression in children, because the potential impact on a child's education and development can be severe and may have serious consequences for the child's future. It is therefore important that all referrals to child psychiatrists should be seen promptly and appropriately.

There are, however, many differences in the way that depression presents in children compared with adults, and also in the way that it is assessed and treated. It is important to be aware of these differences so that childhood depression can be promptly identified, comprehensively assessed and correctly treated. The purpose of this essay is to consider these differences in turn and their implications for mental health services.

Presentation of depression

The maxim of general paediatrics that 'children are not little adults' is equally true when considering mental illness. The concepts involved in depression are often beyond the experience of younger children, and so it is not surprising that they present in a different way from adults.

Children in general have difficulty expressing themselves in 'adult' terms. An adult might talk about their mood or openly complain of feeling 'depressed'. They may also speak (among other things) of a loss of energy, loss of concentration, inability to experience pleasure and hopelessness about the future. However, children may not have developed an understanding of these concepts and so may be unable to articulate how they are feeling in these terms. Instead, they may use their behaviour to express their distress. This may be by becoming withdrawn, unusually quiet and easily upset. Equally, it may appear as increasingly disruptive behaviour and seeking for attention, or in other ways such as school refusal. These symptoms may be an expression of the same underlying feelings as are seen in adults, but in a different way, eg a child with poor concentration may become disruptive in class because they cannot keep their mind on their work.

The context of the presentation may also differ. Adults would be likely to seek help themselves from a family member, the GP or possibly a counselling service. In a severe crisis they might present themselves to the A&E department or perhaps come into contact with the police. Children, on the other hand, are less likely overtly to seek help themselves, and often problems may first present at school. Teachers, educational psychologists and social workers may be the first to become aware of difficulties, although GPs may also be involved if the parents notice problems at home. Depression in children is often related to school, and problems such as school refusal may be the first indicator of difficulties. Similarly, there may be aspects of the school environment (such as bullying) that contribute to the child's difficulties.

Finally, the range of symptoms seen in children will differ from adults. This is at least in part because adults may be better able to verbalise how they are feeling and will respond to questions, whereas children may simply be unable to communicate how they are feeling as effectively. As a result, description of symptoms in children is often based as much (if not more) on observation of behaviour than of reported symptoms. Behavioural change and irritability are both common symptoms of depression in children, but there is a wide range of other symptoms that have been reported.

Assessment of depression

The assessment of depression differs in four main areas between children and adults: the health professionals involved, setting, nature of the assessment and timing of the sessions.

The assessment of depression in adults is usually initially carried out by the GP, who may take on the further management him- or herself or refer to a psychiatrist or a community mental health team. In the last two cases, adult psychiatrists, community psychiatric nurses and other related professionals will become involved and may continue a process of assessment themselves. In children, the school is likely to play a large part in the assessment, and the teacher will often be the first to assess (informally at first) the child's behaviour at school. An educational psychologist may then make a more formal assessment, and a child psychiatrist may often be involved at this point. If the parents raise concerns about the child's behaviour at home, the assessment may go through the GP as described above, although the possibility of a mental illness may not be considered as quickly as a result of the difficulties in presentation described above.

The setting for the assessment is also likely to be different. In adults, the most common setting would be a medical one, such as a GP surgery or a psychiatric outpatient department. Patients may be assessed at home by a psychiatrist or community team, but this depends to a point on the severity of the illness and the urgency of the situation. In children, such a medical setting is less likely to be used. The child may be seen at school or at home, although there is a role for child psychiatry outpatient appointments. These are usually held in a different place to adult appointments, where efforts are made to make the consultation as easy as possible for the child.

The nature of the assessment itself has many differences. In adults, the assessment would take the form of a semi-structured interview with the patient, covering the traditional areas of the psychiatric history. An informant such as a family member would ideally be involved as well. In children the initial assessment is likely to be broader, involving a detailed interview with the parents as well as the child. Information from the school including reports and the views of the teachers may be sought, and observation of the child's behaviour at school by a member of the mental health team might be included.

Finally, the duration of the assessment may be rather longer in children than in adults. The initial assessment in an adult may well be complete after the first interview, and it is usually not necessary to seek information from a number of sources. In children, it may take longer to complete the process of assessment as described above, and a number of sessions with the child or family may be required before a diagnosis can be made. Given that the presentation is relatively non-specific, it may take longer to exclude other possible causes for the presenting problems (such as an underlying physical health problem).

Treatment of depression

As with all mental illness, treatment can be thought of in biological, psychological and social modalities.

Biological (ie drug) treatment for depression is very well established in adults, and there is a very large body of evidence supporting its use. There are many drugs to choose from in a variety of classes, and the recent NICE guidelines for the treatment of depression have provided a clear pathway for approaching treatment. The same is not true for children. Although in theory any of the drugs used in adults could be used in children, there is a much smaller selection of drugs recommended for use. The evidence base is more limited and less rigorous, and the identification and approval of newer medications for use in children are time-consuming and fraught with difficulties. There have been concerns raised recently over the effects of selective serotonin reuptake inhibitors in children, they are no longer recommended for use in this group. Indeed, recent advice from the National Institute of Clinical Health and Excellence (NICE) (2004) has recommended that antidepressants in general should be used only for moderate or severe depression. As a result, using medication in children requires careful consideration and the importance of reaching the correct diagnosis is paramount.

Psychological therapies are of increasing importance in treating depression in all patients. The recent NICE guidelines for the treatment of depression recommends the use of cognitive–behavioural therapy in particular, although there are other well-established approaches including Klerman's (1984) interpersonal therapy and the psychodynamic approach. These treatments have a good evidence base that supports their efficacy. Psychotherapy services are established and in existence, although access to them is often slower than is desirable.

In children, similar therapies can be employed although as with drugs there is less research carried out in this area and therefore less evidence available. It can often be difficult to find therapists willing to take on such work, especially given the pressure on services already with the demand from adult patients. Specialist psychotherapy services for children are few and far between. The success of the therapy depends also on the maturity and development of the child. The main form of therapy used with children (and increasingly with adults) is family therapy in its various forms (behavioural, systemic, etc.). This has the advantage of acknowledging the importance of relationships within the family, and finding ways of helping the whole family to confront the difficulties and find ways of improving them.

Social interventions for depression can vary widely, but again school is a clear point of difference between adults and children. The school environment may be contributing greatly to the child's problems, and unsympathetic staff and bullying from other pupils may be strong perpetuating factors, if not precipitating ones. Hence, a move of school might be an important social intervention with no clear parallel in adults. Housing and financial issues are very important in adults and have an equal impact in children, although the focus will be on the family as a whole rather than on the individual. Clearly, the possibility of domestic conflict and abuse must always be considered (however briefly) when dealing with distressed children.

Implications for practice

There are clearly many differences in all aspects of managing depression in children as opposed to in adults. There are profound implications for mental health services that arise from these.

The many differences in presentation require well-trained staff in both primary and secondary care. GPs, teachers, social workers, parents and children themselves all need to be educated about mental illness, so that it can be identified and treated promptly. Health promotion of this kind is common for physical illness, but almost completely absent for mental illness. The public in general also need to be informed to aid detection and also minimise stigma associated with mental illness. Efforts have already been made in this direction by the Royal College of Psychiatrists with campaigns such as 'Changing Minds'.

The detailed nature of the assessment in children requires a well-trained and well-organised team of all disciplines with good links to schools and Social Services. It is important that assessments are organised rapidly with the minimum amount of disruption, so sufficient resources and appropriate facilities (provision for home visits, suitable consulting rooms, etc.) are also vital.

As with most things, it is not possible to apply what we know of treatment for adults directly to children without modification. All professionals involved need education about which treatments are available and what the indications are for each. More research is needed into drug treatments and appropriate guidelines for their use are required. It is hoped that NICE will deal with this important area without delay. Psychological treatments and especially family therapy have a clear role, but often access to these is not as good as it should be. Greater resources for better access to treatment should be provided.

Conclusion

There are many differences in the presentation, assessment and treatment of depression in children compared with adults, and these have been considered in depth. The potential impact of depression on children and their families is great, and the consequences for the child's future of not identifying and treating it promptly are potentially severe.

There is therefore a continuing need for investment and development of services, along with further research into the treatment of depression in children and a programme of education for the public and professionals alike. It is only by implementing such measures that progress will be made.

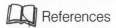 References

Klerman GL et al. *Interpersonal Psychotherapy of Depression*. New York: Basic Books, 1984.

NICE. *Guidelines for Depression*. London: NICE, 2004.

Singleton et al. *Psychiatric Morbidity Among Adults Living in Private Households*. London: Office for National Statistics 2000

US Department of Health and Human Services. *Mental Health: A Report of the Surgeon General*. US Department of Health and Human Services, 1999.

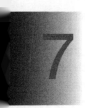

Part II:
patient management
problems

Introduction

The PMP section of the Part II examination takes the form of a single half-hour-long interview during which you will discuss three clinical scenarios with the examiners. This forms part of the clinical day in Part II. It may be held before or after the Individual Patient Assessment (IPA) but you will be sent the timetable in advance.

PMP is short for 'Patient Management Problem' and, for each of the three PMPs in the exam, you will be given a brief description of a clinical scenario on a piece of paper. The description from the piece of paper will be read out to you and you are expected to listen in silence. A series of questions, also known as probes, will follow, allowing the examiners to assess your understanding of the situation and your approach to it.

The first examiner will ask you about the first PMP, while the second examiner sits quietly. The second examiner will then ask you questions about the second PMP and then the first examiner will question you again about the third PMP. There are three PMPs in total, in 30 minutes, allocated 10 minutes each. There is no discretion with regard to timing, so exactly 10 minutes will be spent on each PMP, regardless of your performance.

The PMP is not a test of factual knowledge – it is designed to assess your ability to cope with a range of potentially difficult situations in the most appropriate manner. The questions are standardised across the country so that every candidate taking part in the PMPs at the same time will be asked the same questions. This represents significant progress over the situation not so many years ago when examiners maintained their own collections of PMPs and could ask whatever they wanted!

Revision techniques

Very little additional factual knowledge is required for the PMP section of the examination beyond what you have already learnt for the ISQ/EMI section of the written paper, the essay paper and the long case.

The most important difference between the PMPs and the other parts of the examination is that you are required to talk about your findings rather than writing about them. Unlike the long case, you will have no time to prepare a presentation. You will have to answer the questions put to you immediately and will have very little time to think. Anxiety will be high in the exam and you should aim to cover all the common types of PMP in your revision, so that you can identify the important themes in any given PMP in the real exam. This will allow you to minimise the thinking that you have to do, and will ensure that you appear polished and ready.

These facts have important implications for your revision schedule. The most important revision you can do for the PMP consists of getting together with a group of other candidates and practising PMPs with them. Take it in turns to ask questions and to answer them. As with the group revision techniques for the ISQs and EMIs, this will maximise your revision time and make sure that you learn as efficiently as possible, as well as increasing your motivation when you're tired, or not feeling strongly inclined to work for any other reason.

You should get hold of as many practice PMPs as possible and practise these as much as you can in your revision group. There is little point in making anything other than brief notes on PMPs as you are required to talk about the answers rather than write them down. You should talk about the PMPs often in your revision group and get as much practice as possible.

As mentioned above, the examiners are looking for evidence that you can handle potentially difficult situations in a calm and ordered manner. An example of a PMP might be as follows:

> You receive a referral from a GP who is asking you to assess a 13-year-old boy who may have an autistic spectrum disorder. How will you assess and manage this patient?

It is important to remember that this is not a test of your detailed knowledge of the clinical features, epidemiology, natural history and prognosis of autistic spectrum disorders. That was assessed in the ISQ/EMI paper. The PMPs are a test of your knowledge of how such a situation might be managed.

It is very important with PMPs to start with the absolute basics. There is no one right answer to the PMP given above, but a good start would be to say that you would first ask the GP for more information, such as the reasons why they consider the patient to have an autistic spectrum disorder, details of any previous contact with psychiatric services, as well as any previous contact with other medical specialities. It will then be appropriate to discuss the patient with your multidisciplinary team at a referrals meeting or other weekly meeting, such as the ward round or multidisciplinary team meeting. Stress the importance of the multidisciplinary aspects of the assessment that are vital in this case. You should then say that you would arrange to see the patient along with his parents or carers in your outpatient clinic if possible. Again, sticking to the absolute basics, you should send the patient a letter, inviting him or her and a family member to attend the clinic, explaining the purpose of visit and who will be present at the interview, as well as how long the interview will take, directions to the hospital, as well as information about parking or public transport. You should also make arrangements to search the hospital records to see if this patient has been seen previously as well as informing your colleagues at your weekly meeting of the planned assessment. You should indicate very strongly that it is important to assess the patient in a range of settings, including at school and at home as well as in the clinic. Invite one of your nursing colleagues to attend the initial interview where you can introduce them to the patient and his or her family and inform them that this nurse will be seeing the patient at home and perhaps at school, if they are agreeable.

It is necessary to talk about the features that you would be looking for, particularly in the initial interview, with particular reference to the ICD-10 criteria for the disorder in question. What you should avoid doing is talking in detail through each of the criteria in turn because this will simply take too long and dominate the 10 minutes that you have for this PMP. You should, however, spend enough time talking about the main features so that the examiners know that you understand the nature of the disorder and would be able to recognise it. You should then stress the importance of obtaining a collateral history from a relative or carer, and stress that this does not need to be done in the initial interview. At the end of the initial interview, you would explain to the patient and the carer/parent that members of your team would very much like to see the patient at home and at school to continue with the assessment.

After the interview, you should discuss the case with members of your team and arrange for your nursing colleague, and perhaps a social worker, to visit the family home, having established that this is safe, to continue the assessment. On this visit, the team will be looking for any differences in presentation between the clinic and the home, as well as getting more detailed information from family members about the course of the problems to date and what the particular difficulties are at the present time. A visit to the school should include discussions with teachers who know the patient well, and information from old school reports about any particular difficulties experienced. It is also important to establish whether the patient has a statement of special educational need.

Having gathered all the necessary information, you should arrange a case conference, inviting the whole range of professionals involved in the case, including the patient's general practitioner, to discuss the case in detail and come to an agreement about a diagnosis. It is also vitally important to devise a management plan to discuss how any problems can be addressed. This should be based on the most significant problems at the time of the assessment as well as any problems that can be predicted for the future.

It is then important to explain this diagnosis to the patient and the patient's carer in terms that they can understand, while supplying them with written information that they can refer to afterwards. A follow-up visit from the nurse may be helpful in explaining this further. Any management plan that has been made should be implemented and further review in the outpatient clinic and at home should be arranged to ensure that the expected support is given and the expected progress made.

This PMP illustrates some of the common features of PMPs, including the need to start with absolute basics, such as the sending out of appointment letters, and making arrangements to see patients in certain places, such as outpatient clinics or at home. In discussing cases informally with your colleagues at work, you would take these basics for granted but it is important to mention them in PMPs because it demonstrates that you have experience of such situations and knowledge of how healthcare systems operate. If you miss out details such as the sending of appointment letters, the examiners will interrupt you to ask how you would arrange the appointment and this is likely to shake your confidence and impair your performance.

Particularly important in PMPs are such things as multidisciplinary working, case conferences, assessment in a variety of settings, details about when and how to assess people and issues of safety. If a PMP involves the assessment of somebody in prison, it is important to say that you would contact the prison in advance to arrange your visit, ask what forms of identification are required to gain access to the prison and suggest that it might be useful to telephone the prison on the day of the assessment to ensure that the prisoner/patient is still there and that the prison personnel are still aware of the exact time of your visit. You will also need to inform the prison in advance if any other member of your team will be accompanying you. If you have visited prisons, you will be aware of these issues, even if you take them for granted, but you must mention them in the PMP.

What do you should do in a PMP is try to remember exactly what would be done in the real world and communicate this to the examiners. In reality, the secretary probably writes and sends appointment letters, and you may never have seen one, but you need to mention the appointment letter in the PMP. The difference between the world of the

PMP and the real world is that, in the world of the PMP, you always have a full multidisciplinary team at your disposal, with almost limitless amounts of time in which to assess and manage people. In reality, you may work in a service where some member of a multidisciplinary team is persistently absent from work with sickness or where a certain post is unfilled; this obviously limits the effectiveness of the team and hampers assessments. This is never the case in the world of the PMP. Some candidates have been reported to have said such things as 'we have no psychologist on our team, so I would not be able to pursue a referral' – you should avoid repeating this mistake at all costs!

The ideal answer to a PMP consists of you starting to talk after the first question is asked and continuing to talk, answering the examiners' questions before they have asked them, for the rest of the 10 minutes. Needless to say, this never happens in practice and you will usually be interrupted at some point, and asked further questions.

Although you must talk about the basics, as outlined above, you should not use this as a means of stalling for time or trying to delay talking about the real issues. It is not necessary to talk in great detail about exactly what questions you would ask in the history. You should stress that, in taking a history from a patient with a depressive disorder, for example, you would focus particularly on features of depressive disorders such as low mood, biological features of depression and features indicating a risk of self-harm or suicide. What you should not do is say that you would start by asking the patient's name, address, date of birth, current age, civil status, accommodation details, and so on, before talking about their current problems, then going on to talk about how these problems have developed over the past few years, etc. This sort of excessive detail will irritate the examiners and give the impression that you are playing for time so you do not have to answer difficult questions later on about investigation, management and prognosis.

As with the other parts of the examination, such as ISQs and EMIs, some areas are covered more commonly in the PMP examination than others. Particular favourites include emergency situations such as an inpatient threatening staff or other patients with a weapon such as a knife. This scenario requires you to make sure that staff and other patients are as safe as possible without confronting the person with the weapon. It is vitally important to state that you would dial 999 to seek police assistance as soon as possible and that the only people who are capable of confronting an armed person safely are the police. You will fail this PMP if you describe heroic courses of action such as negotiating with the patient, entering the room with the patient to talk to him or her or trying to persuade the patient to give up the weapon.

Try getting hold of as many PMP practice books as possible and practising them with your colleagues. Using the model answers given in the books; you will quickly learn about the most common scenarios and the important areas that need to be covered in your answers.

After you have passed the written part of the examination, and start revising in earnest for the clinical, it is very important that you arrange as many practice PMP sessions with senior colleagues as possible before the clinical exam. Try to ensure that these practice PMP sessions are as realistic as possible, with two examiners taking turns to ask questions and 10-minute time limits for each PMP. You should try to have three PMPs per session. What you will find is that the process is quite tiring and you often feel that you have made mistakes on the first or second PMP and have difficulty concentrating on the next PMP as a result. This will happen in the real exam and it is important to experience this beforehand so that you can develop your own coping strategies. Many people believe that they have failed the first or second PMP and simply feel like walking out of the room rather than continuing. In many cases, however, they have actually done rather well, so it is important that you continue with the process regardless of your perception of your performance.

Exam techniques

If you have practised the PMPs with colleagues, you will know exactly what to expect in the real exam, which will make the experience considerably less difficult.

When the PMP scenario is being read out to you, you will have a copy of it in your hands. There is no need to write anything at all during this time, or at any other point in the interview. All the information that you need is presented to you on a sheet of paper and you do not need to write anything. Some candidates do feel the need to write, and it mystifies the examiners as well as looking unnecessary and potentially concerning.

It is important to control your anxiety in the exam and to remember that you should answer questions by starting with the most simple and most common things before moving on to more complex areas. As you have experienced at medical school, you will be asked about the investigations that you would like to carry out to investigate certain presentations, such as psychosis. It is vitally important to mention blood tests such as full blood count, urea and electrolytes, etc. first, before going on to talk about advanced imaging techniques if required. If you fail to control your anxiety and simply say the first thing that comes into your head, such as 'an MRI scan' for the investigation of psychosis, you will find yourself answering very difficult questions about the details of changes in cerebral structure that have been found on neuroimaging in patients with psychosis. It is far better to start with the basics, about which you can answer questions relatively easily. It is likely that you will never then get on to the discussion of neuroimaging, as time will run out, so you can avoid the more difficult areas altogether.

When discussing investigations, try to avoid talking about 'routine' blood tests. This gives the impression that you would carry out all these blood tests on all your patients, without thinking. Although this may be true, you do not want to give the examiners this impression and you are very likely to be asked why you would perform, for example, a test of the sodium level in someone presenting with auditory hallucinations. It is better to present a brief justification for the blood tests at the same time as you tell the examiners which blood tests you would like to order. This gives the impression that you have thought about which tests to conduct and have tailored them to the individual patient. It is also preferably to use the full name for the test, for example, 'liver function tests' rather than 'LFTs'. After discussing the history and mental state examination, you might say:

> In the initial investigation of a patient presenting with a first episode of psychosis, I would arrange blood tests to exclude the possibility of a contributing organic disorder. Full blood count should be carried out to exclude conditions such as anaemia or acute infection, a test of urea and electrolytes would exclude hyponatraemia or other electrolyte disturbance as a contributory cause. Liver function tests might indicate excessive alcohol consumption or other physical problems.

This indicates that you are aware that it is unlikely that anything detected by these blood tests is causing the symptoms, but that it is important to be aware that there may be a contributory organic cause that needs to be identified and treated. Examiners will have a difficult time criticising you for this position, although they may have some questions. You have also spoken intelligently for quite a proportion of the total time allowed for the PMP, so there is less time available for difficult questions. A less appropriate answer might be:

> I would organise routine blood tests, including full blood count, U&Es, LFTs, TFTs, CRP and ESR.

Not only is this full of acronyms, but you are also leaving yourself open to questions about what proportion of people with auditory hallucinations have an elevated CRP, why you think the ESR might be raised, and whether you would arrange LFTs on every patient being admitted and whether this is justifiable.

A common mistake (throughout medical school as well as postgraduate exams) is to mention a rare or unlikely disease or investigation. When asked about possible organic causes for psychosis, mention substance misuse or systemic illness first, rather than Wilson's disease or another relatively uncommon condition. If you do mention a rare disorder such as this, be prepared for difficult questions about serum copper levels, exotic diagnostic tests, etc. Keep it simple!

You will often be asked how you would assess and manage certain situations. The correct answer is always that you would take a full history and conduct a full mental state examination, before carrying out basic investigations and seeking collateral information such as reports from carers, relatives, friends, schools, police, GPs, inpatient staff, hospital records, etc. Obtaining collateral information is a vital part of the answer to almost any PMP.

If you are presented with an emergency situation, such as the PMP outlined above involving an armed patient on a ward, you must still obtain collateral information from the nursing staff, even if this takes only 30 seconds. You might want to know if the patient is known to be intoxicated or if he or she has delusions or other concerns about a particular member of staff for a fellow patient. You do not want to know this so that you can intervene and manage the situation, but so that this vital information can be passed on to the police as soon as they arrive. Generally, the more time you have to manage a situation, the more collateral information you will obtain.

PMPs based on learning disability scenarios are a special case, because the usual range of precipitating factors has to be considered, although there is special emphasis on the possibilities of organic problems, environmental changes and abuse by carers.

The examiners are given three 'probes' that indicate further questions that they should ask after the initial scenario and introductory questions. These 'probes' were introduced in an effort to standardise PMPs across the various centres and to prevent examiners going off on tangents or asking irrelevant questions. Once the areas indicated by the three 'probes' have been covered, however, no guidance is available to the examiners and they will be forced to think of further areas of discussion. This can be difficult if one examiner has a specific area of interest or wants to lead the discussion along an unusual or difficult path. In the worst case, you can be left playing a game of 'guess what I'm thinking' with the examiners, when they ask questions with a specific answer in mind that you are struggling to provide. Although you may already have demonstrated enough knowledge to pass by this stage, it can be an uncomfortable situation.

If you can talk intelligently and at some length about the opening question and the three subsequent 'probes', you can pass the PMP without venturing into the examiner-specific territory that follows. Although difficult to achieve in practice, this should be something to aim for.

Something to avoid at any cost is arguing with the examiners. This will always count against you and you should not aim to be in disagreement with the two people who are marking you. Even if the examiners tell you something that you believe to be factually inaccurate or just plain wrong, do not argue! Look it up afterwards and discuss it with your friends, but do not dispute it with the examiners in the exam. Many candidates have 'failed with their boots on' by arguing with the examiners about a minor point, when they could have passed by ignoring this and talking about something else.

8 Part II: the long case

Introduction

The Part II clinical is an important part of the overall Part II exam. It marks the final hurdle before you are granted membership of the Royal College of Psychiatrists. By this stage you will be experienced in a range of psychiatric subspecialties. Having passed the written component of the Part II, you have demonstrated that you possess the factual knowledge required by the College. The Part II clinical is largely a test of clinical skill and technique.

If you fail the clinical exam, you face the unenviable task of re-sitting the written exam. As you will know by now, preparation for this is time-consuming and difficult. Your preparation for, and performance during, the clinical exam is therefore of paramount importance.

Preparation for the long case

As with all clinical exams, preparation is the key to success in the long case, or the 'individual patient assessment' (IPA), as it is referred to by the Royal College. You will have no time to 'think on your feet' during the exam itself, so you must make sure that you are fully prepared and ready for all eventualities. Preparation must focus on technique rather than on amassing further factual knowledge. In this part of the exam more than any other, there are ways to maximise your chances of success on the day itself.

Your preparation should start with a thorough understanding of the format and requirements of the exam. You must travel to an unfamiliar and often distant hospital, frequently staying locally the night before the exam, where you are put into a room with a real patient and given 1 hour to take a full history and conduct relevant mental state and physical examinations. After this time, you are taken to a room with two examiners (and possibly a Royal College observer) and must give a short presentation of your findings, lasting approximately 8 minutes. This should include a brief introduction, history, mental state and physical examinations, differential diagnosis and preferred diagnosis. The examiners will then invite you to bring the patient into the room and ask the patient about two specific aspects of the history again, in front of the examiners. This is called the observed interview and it lasts 10 minutes. After this, you will show the patient out of the room and the examiners will have a further 10 minutes to ask you a range of questions about the patient, the diagnosis or differential diagnosis, and any other subjects that they consider relevant. After this final ordeal, you are free to go.

A list of presentations

The first step in preparing for the long case is to draw up a list of the possible presentations that you might be faced with in the real exam, which can then be developed into lists of key points to look out for in the history and examination for each of these presentations. It is useful to base your preparation on the general type of presentation rather than a specific diagnosis because it is unlikely that the patient will say 'I have bipolar disorder' at the start of the interview (although this does happen!). You are likely to become aware quite quickly of the general type of disorder, if not the precise diagnosis. It should be obvious whether you are seeing someone with psychosis or with an eating disorder, for example, in the first few minutes of the interview. The list of presentations might include:

- Forgetfulness in old age

- Substance misuse

- Psychosis

- Affective disorder

- Neurosis

- Eating disorder

- Disorders relating to childbirth

- Personality disorder

- Learning difficulty

- Developmental disorder.

For each of these presentations, you should then prepare an outline template for the history and mental state and physical examinations, including questions to ask and positive signs and symptoms, as well as any important negative findings. This should be broken down according to your own method of history taking. A standard format might include the following.

Standard template/format for history taking – for each individual presentation

Demographic information

The patient's name is critical. Burn this into your memory! You will be starting your presentation to the examiners with this and it will not look good if you can't remember it or are not sure how to pronounce it. If in doubt, ask the patient.

Date of birth (and therefore age), gender, employment, type of accommodation (flat, house, private, rented or local authority) are all vital. Civil status (married, single, cohabiting), is also important and a good question is 'Who else is at home with you?' followed by 'What is your relationship with them?'. These are non-threatening, non-judgemental questions that will throw light on the patient's domestic situation. It is important to know the patient's sexual orientation. This usually becomes obvious during the course of the history, but you must clarify this with the patient if you are still unsure by the time you reach the end of the history.

It is also important to establish whether the patient is an inpatient or an outpatient and the name of the consultant in charge of his or her care. If the patient is being treated as an inpatient, which ward/unit is he or she on and when was he or she admitted? Has he or she moved wards/units in the meantime, eg from an acute unit to a rehabilitation unit? If being followed up in the community, what sort of team is looking after the patient – early intervention, assertive outreach, drug and alcohol services, forensic services or a generic community mental health team?

Presenting complaint with duration

This should take the form of 'Mr Smith presents with a history of low mood/hallucinations/anxiety in public places for the last 3 weeks/3 months'.

Although this sounds easy, it is absolutely critical that an appropriate duration is given for the presenting complaint. A successful history depends on establishing the duration of the presenting complaint, as everything before the date given as the start of the presenting complaint must be covered in the past psychiatric history. In the next part of the history (history of presenting complaint), you must give full details of the patient's course, symptoms, coping strategies, etc., beginning from the time you identify as the start of the presenting complaint. In your short presentation to the examiners, you will be expected to identify predisposing, precipitating and maintaining factors, and these must all relate to the current episode. Predisposing factors must have been present long before the current episode started. Precipitating factors must have been present just before the current episode and maintaining factors must have continued during the current episode.

You can appreciate that defining the start of the current episode, the duration of the presenting complaint, is vital. How should you decide it?

It is ideally marked by the start of the current episode of active symptoms. This may be easy to identify, in the case of someone with a current episode of hypomania dating back 3 weeks in the context of bipolar disorder. It is very easy to identify in a woman with postpartum psychosis. It can be difficult in patients with chronic disorders such as obsessive–compulsive disorder. You must decide for yourself what an appropriate duration of presenting complaint should be and then base your interview on this information.

The real danger here lies in identifying the presenting complaint as starting more than 6 months ago. You will then have too much work to do in taking the history of the presenting complaint. In a straightforward case of a recurrent depressive disorder, you will have to cover low mood, insomnia, loss of interests, poor appetite, decreased energy, loss of confidence, guilt, thoughts of self-harm, poor concentration and psychomotor retardation. It is reasonable to get some feeling for how all of these have developed over the last few weeks or even months, but impossible to trace their development over 3 or 4 years, in any detail. If you set the history or presenting complaint too early, you will have too much to do.

History of presenting complaint

Look at your list of presentations and draw up a list of possible ICD-10 diagnoses for each, eg the presentation 'Affective disorder' might include:

- Hypomania
- Mania (with/without psychosis)
- Bipolar affective disorder
- Depressive episode (mild/moderate/severe)
- Recurrent depressive disorder

- Cyclothymia

- Dysthymia.

Then make sure that in your standard interview template for 'Affective disorders' you have a list of all the questions needed to cover the ICD-10 criteria for each of these disorders. When you then ask these questions, you have already got a good structure, you have established a firm diagnosis according to ICD-10 and you have made yourself more aware of what the ICD-10 criteria are.

It is also important to ask about what help the patient has sought. Did he ring up the consultant's secretary and make an appointment when the patient realised that he was becoming unwell? Did he hide upstairs when the mental health team can to see him at home? Did he see his GP or was he paranoid about her? What does he think about that now?

You should ask about the effect that the symptoms have had on the patient. What do his family/employers/friends think about the situation? What does the patient find to be the greatest problem? If he could change one thing about his current condition, what would it be? What would he like to be done about his problems? These questions give you an understanding of the patient's insight into his illness but they also demonstrate to the examiners that you are able to see the patient as a real person, rather than as a collection of signs and symptoms.

Family history

This should include parental ages (or ages at death and causes of death), and parental occupations as well as number and order of siblings. Any family history of mental disorder should be noted, along with treatment and course.

Personal history

This must clearly be tailored to the individual patient and is dependent to some extent on the patient's age. Details of the schooling of a dementing 83-year-old man may be relevant, but not in as much detail as in the case of a 17-year-old woman with social phobia. It is important to cover aspects such as the following:

- The patient's mother's health during pregnancy

- Birth complications

- Ill-health during infancy and childhood

- Difficulties at home during childhood (financial, social, alcohol- or drug-related, violence, abuse, neglect, etc.)

- Any difficulties in early relationships with close family members

- Schooling: type and locations of schools, academic and social performance, disciplinary problems, suspensions and expulsions

- Social activity during adolescence

- Qualifications on leaving school

- Employment history

- Accommodation and co-habitees.

There is a lot of material here that needs to be covered. Any patient over the age of 30 presents a challenge in terms of timing. There is not enough time to cover all these areas in great detail. The precise start and finish dates of each of the patient's 27 jobs are unimportant. You should aim to get across an impression of the patient's history. Did he leave most of his jobs after a fight with a colleague? Has he generally stayed in jobs for years on end or has he changed jobs every 2 months? Why has he been unemployed for the past 2 years after a lifetime of regular employment. Be alert for progressive changes such as a slow deterioration in the quality of jobs that the patient has held, or progressively less successful or shorter jobs. Any sudden or marked changes need to be explained. Why did the patient move from a privately owned four-bedroom house to a council flat after 18 years?

Sometimes, the patient may refuse to talk about certain areas, or may be evasive and vague, despite clear, patient and repeated clarification. This is not your fault and is certainly not a weakness. Tell the examiners that you were keen to know about the patient's most recent job/use of alcohol, etc., but that the patient was unwilling to go into detail. Many candidates will simply ignore this issue and hope that the examiners will not notice the lack of a full history, but what you are doing in reporting a reluctance to discuss a certain area is noting an important aspect of the mental state. This is a strength and not something that you should hide.

Past medical history

Important medical conditions (epilepsy, diabetes, cardiovascular disease, arthritis, etc.) should be covered here, as well as any surgery that the patient has undergone.

History of alcohol and substance misuse

Taking a history of alcohol and substance misuse should be second nature by this stage, but candidates have failed on this point in the recent past. Detail is important here and the CAGE questions (see page 32) are not sufficient. Ask about the strengths (in terms of alcohol by volume) of any drinks taken, when the patient has his first drink of the day and specifically about symptoms of withdrawal. It is important to know how much the patient is spending on illicit drugs and where the money is coming from, as well as the context of their use – on their own, with others or only after arguments?

Forensic history

Has the patient been in trouble with the police? Was he charged with anything or convicted of anything? Did he receive a community or a custodial sentence? Did he comply with this?

Past psychiatric history

The past psychiatric history is exactly that – what has happened in the past. It ends at the time that you have given as the start of the history of the presenting complaint.

It is clear that very different points will be relevant for an eating disorder presentation compared with a presentation of schizophrenia. You should discuss your outline history with your friends and colleagues as part of your ongoing revision group and make sure that they are as comprehensive as possible. There may not be time in the actual exam to present all of your positive and negative findings, but there will be time during the hour that you have with the patient to ask all the relevant questions, and, armed with a full knowledge of the patient, you can choose what to present and what to leave out.

By the end of the history taking, you should be in a position to draw up a list of differential diagnoses, classified according to ICD-10 criteria. Again, these should be part of your standard templates as they are relatively easy to list for each of the main presentation types. An example would be a patient giving a history of depressive symptoms. Depending on the specifics of the history, the differential diagnosis might include:

- A single episode of depressive disorder
- Recurrent depressive disorder
- Bipolar affective disorder
- Adjustment disorder

- Schizoaffective disorder

- Organic disorder.

It is important that you always include a sensible organic cause as part of your differential diagnosis because this demonstrates that you are aware that organic causes need to be excluded. If it is very unlikely that an organic cause is the source of the problems, then feel free to say so, but you must mention one anyway. A useful phrase here is 'This diagnosis must be considered, if only so that it can be excluded'. Endocrine abnormalities can account for a wide range of psychiatric presentations.

Relationship history

It is important to get some basic information about the patient's relationships. The detail required will vary according to the relevance of relationships to the history of mental health difficulties, but you should know the patient's age at first relationship, approximate number and length of relationships, as well as factors causing relationships to end, and what maintained the relationships. Were they founded on shared use of illicit substances or a love of opera? It is important to find out if the patient has been involved in sexual relationships. You should then have enough information to determine the patient's sexual orientation, but if you do not, ask the patient.

Mental state examination

Having decided on your differential diagnoses, you should conduct the mental state examination (MSE) with the specific aim of confirming your chosen diagnosis. The MSE can therefore be tailored to the individual presentation.

You should again draw up a list of areas to be covered in the MSE that are specific to the individual presentation. It is important that you are familiar with this section in the exam because most of the information in the MSE section can be gleaned as you take the history. There simply will not be time to conduct a full, separate MSE. Certain aspects of the MSE, such as orientation and Mini-Mental State Examination, can be carried out at the relevant point in the history or at the end of the history.

The standard format for the MSE is as follows:

- Appearance and behaviour

- Mood

- Speech

- Thought

- Perception

- Cognition

- Insight.

You may have developed your own format for the MSE in your own practice, but may want to adopt the above for exam purposes so that you do not appear to the examiners to be idiosyncratic and therefore potentially concerning.

Physical examination

After the MSE comes the physical examination. The importance of this cannot be overstated. It is often neglected, particularly during the stage of preparation for the Part II clinical, but it is important to remember that it attracts as many marks as the MSE. Again, you must have an outline format for the physical examination, for each of the presentations that you have identified above. We would suggest the following format for a physical examination:

- Pulse

- Blood pressure

- Temperature

- Signs of jaundice, anaemia, clubbing, cyanosis, oedema and lymphadenopathy, and hepatic disease

- Hand signs including tremor, nail biting, palmar erythema and nicotine staining

- Head and neck signs including enophthalmos, exophthalmos, goitre and the quality of the skin, including dryness or oiliness

- Weight and height may be relevant if body mass index needs to be calculated.

It is vital to look out for the occasional surprises. You will feel very foolish if you fail to comment on the patient's artificial limb, eye or other prosthesis. It is also very important to state the obvious. If the patient has a prominent scar or pigmented lesion, comment on this. As long as you do so in a professional manner, you will not be criticised for lack of empathy. With elderly patients, signs of normal ageing such as arcus senilis should be commented on.

Further details of history taking, as well as mental and physical state examination, are given in *A Guide to Psychiatric Examination* by Drs Aquilina and Warner. Many other books cover this area but are aimed mainly at physicians, and these often go into too much detail for the MRCPsych.

During the process of making your standard templates for the different diagnoses, you will refine your own format for history taking, as well as mental and physical state examinations. The precise details of your own individual format do not matter but it is important that you use a format with which the examiners will feel comfortable, because you do not want to appear difficult or unusual on the day.

Having prepared these templates and practised the questions that you will ask, it is important that you are aware of how you must present the summary of your findings to the examiners. You are given 10 minutes to present this information but it is best practice to use approximately 7 or 8 minutes of this time actually to present. This allows time for getting in and out of the room as well as brief introductions. The most important part of your presentation is the opening sentence.

If you appear dysfluent or hesitant you will immediately give the examiners a bad impression. Regardless of marking schemes and the supposed objectivity of exams, first impressions do make a difference and you must get off to a professional and impressive start. Your first sentence should be a brief statement about the patient, including their age, gender, name, type of accommodation, civil status and occupation. An example might be:

> 'I have been speaking to Mr Smith, a 37-year-old man living in a two-bedroom council flat with his wife and two children. He currently works as a labourer in a warehouse.'

Again, the exact wording of this introductory statement can vary according to your own personal preference and to the patient with whom you are presented. It is important that you decide on your own style before the exam and practise even this apparently simple task with as many people as possible. You should then move on fluently to the presentation itself and you should practise often enough so that you can judge the time taken to present quite accurately with only occasional glances at your watch.

Having presented the history and MSE, it is critical of that you also present the physical state examination. As has already been mentioned, this carries as many marks as the MSE but is an area that is often neglected by candidates. For this reason it is particularly important because a good physical state examination will really make you stand out from the crowd. You must cover the basics such as pulse, blood pressure and any other important positive or negative signs relevant to the presentations with which you are faced. It is simply not acceptable to omit these fundamental aspects of the physical examination and you will be marked down very heavily if you do.

After you have decided on the individual format for your own history, MSE and physical state examination, you should ensure that all of the specific presentation types on your list of possible presentations conform to this one style. You will refine them during your revision but you should be happy with them at least two weeks before the actual clinical exam. We would suggest that you simply practise the history taking and examination after this time, with as many of your friends, registrars and consultants as possible. This is critical to your success in the exam and often makes the difference between passing and failing. It is important that you practise with as many people as possible and that you present to people you find anxiety provoking so that you are exposed to as much anxiety as possible. This will of course reduce the level of anxiety that you feel in the actual exam, which will benefit you enormously. It is particularly important to present to consultants whom you do not know well or who have a reputation for being difficult, because this is as close to the real exam situation as it is possible to get.

Each of the people with whom you practise will give you different advice about how to structure the history and examination and how to present. It is important that you listen to them and be prepared to change your format to some extent, but you will inevitably be given different advice by every different person with whom you practise. Do not try to please them all, because this is impossible. It is important that you present in a competent and practised manner but there is no one ideal way to present that will guarantee success. It is important that you are happy with your own style of presentation.

The observed interview comes next and there is very little specific preparation that you can do for this part of the exam. It may be helpful to list the subjects that you might be expected to discuss and these include:

- Alcohol or illicit drug consumption

- Depressive symptoms

- Thoughts of suicide or self-harm

- Hallucinatory experiences

- Relationship issues

- Fear of fatness

- Symptoms of elevated mood

- Obsessional or compulsive symptoms

- Frontal lobe signs

- Memory impairment

- Risk assessment.

Anything that is particularly prominent in the history may be asked about. One topic of conversation among trainees is the idea that you can steer the examiners towards certain topics, which you have prepared in advance. This is underhand and could backfire, but the idea discussed is that you can take a good alcohol history, for example, and then tell the examiners that you did not have time to discuss the patient's use of alcohol in great detail.

You may wish to develop your own standard format for each of these eventualities, or just for the ones that you personally find difficult.

The final part of the exam is the general question and answer session. This is very varied and can include specific factual questions as well as more general discussion of a wide range of subjects relevant to psychiatry. It is best seen as a test of a wider knowledge and you will have covered the vast majority of information required in your successful preparation for the written part of the exam.

The day of the exam

Nothing should be left to chance on the day of the actual exam. You will be sitting the exam in another part of the country and in most cases you will be arriving in the local area the night before. It is worth spending some money on a decent hotel where you can have a good night's sleep before the exam. You should make sure that you know where the exam is being held and preferably drive to the venue the day before the actual exam to make sure that you can find it and that you know how long the journey takes.

Allow plenty of time to arrive at the venue because arriving late will almost guarantee that you fail the exam. Once in the venue, the main job will be to calm your nerves.

The initial interview

When the long case exam starts, you will be given some blank pieces of paper and shown into the interview room. Make good use of this time by writing the headings from your standard templates on the blank paper before the patient is shown in. This is not cheating and will allow you to start promptly when the patient arrives.

It is critical that you establish a good rapport with the patient as quickly as possible after the initial introduction. Explain to the patient that this is an exam situation and that you are very nervous. Apologise in advance in case you appear brusque or anxious. Reassure the patient that you are being examined rather than them. In some cases, the patient may tell you their diagnosis and outline their history in an appropriate fashion. If this happens, you are very lucky and should take advantage of this situation. Do make sure that you conduct a full history in any case as the patient is unlikely to present you with every piece of information in the order that suits you best.

Take your history, noting any relevant aspects of the mental state examination as you proceed in order to save time at the end. Try to write on only one side of the paper because this will minimise the shuffling of paper in front of the examiners. Aim to finish your interview approximately 15 minutes before the hour is over and then start on the physical examination. You can ask further questions during the physical examination if you need to.

Having finished the physical examination, you should review your notes and ask any questions that you forgot earlier. This last 10 minutes of the hour is crucial and you are likely to remember important points. On no account ask the patient to leave before the full hour is over. Do not rewrite your notes at this stage as this is too time-consuming but feel free to annotate them and add to them if necessary.

At the end of the interview, it is vital that you again thank the patient profusely for his or her help and support at this difficult time for you. Explain that you will be seeing him or her again in approximately 10 minutes in front of the examiners and that this is once again very stressful and difficult for you. Reassure the patient that he or she is not being examined and thank him or her again for his or her time.

The patient will then be shown from the room and you will be taken to a waiting room outside the main exam. Use this time to prepare your short presentation, particularly the introduction, which needs to be fluent and spoken from memory, rather than read from a sheet. Gather your thoughts and prepare yourself for the examiners.

The case presentation

Once you are in the exam room, adopt a posture with which you are comfortable and sit as still as you can. You should have written on only one side of the paper, so there will be no need to turn pages over; you can simply slide them behind each other when you need to move to the next page and this looks much more professional and practised.

The examiners will often ask you to tell them about the patient, up to the stage of the physical examination, or differential diagnosis. You should stop at this point and expect to be questioned about the remaining subjects, such as investigations, management or prognosis.

The observed interview

The examiners will ask you to invite the patient in for the observed interview. You should make sure that there are sufficient chairs, particularly if the patient is accompanied by a carer. Plan the route before you invite the patient into the room. Are there any rugs that she may trip over? Is there enough space for a Zimmer frame or wheelchair? If the patient has told you to call her by a first name, tell the examiners this before you invite her in because you do not want to appear inappropriate or over-familiar.

When you have brought the patient in, thank her again for her time and reassure her that you are being examined rather than her. Introduce her to the examiners, but do not feel that you need to remember the names of the examiners. Ask the patient's permission to ask questions again, reminding her that you mentioned that you would like to ask her questions again. Tell her that you may have discussed some of these questions before, but that the examiners would like to listen to the interview. Take the history as you have been instructed by the examiners and move on to the second subject after approximately 5 minutes when you have covered the first subject appropriately.

When you have covered the whole history to your satisfaction and have spent approximately 10 minutes doing so, thank the patient very much for her time and escort her from the room. The examiners will not want to intervene to tell you to move on after 5 minutes, or to end the interview after 10 minutes, so do not wait for them to indicate that you have done enough.

Close the door behind you after you have shown the patient out. Make sure that you show her back to the waiting room or to the area where the exam assistant is waiting for her because you do not want to be seen abandoning her in an unfamiliar corridor. Thank the patient again for her time and tell her that you have now finished and will not be seeing her again.

The question and answer session

When you return to the exam room for the final question-and-answer session, knock on the door and enter when instructed. You are now nearing the final part of the long case exam and the ordeal is nearly over.

You must simply answer the questions as best you can and, at any cost, avoid arguing with the examiners, even if you think that they are wrong.

Conclusion

The individual patient assessment, or long case, is one of the most demanding parts of the MRCPsych exam. It requires careful preparation, planning, concentration, tact, factual knowledge and close attention to timing.

This part of the exam remains the one where chance plays the largest role, because patients can be unpredictable, but, with the appropriate revision, as well as care on the day, you will improve your chances of being successful.

Index

absolute benefit increase (ABI) 58
acetylcholine receptors 21
actors, in OSCE 36–7
β_1-adrenoceptors 21
affective disorders 152–3
alcohol consumption, and exams 4
alcohol misuse
    ICD–10 criteria for dependence 32, 33
    and long case 155
    and OSCE 30, 32, 33
Allport, G. 25
antipsychotic-induced pyrexia 15
antipsychotics, atypical 111–13
anxiety, and exams 4
areas of weakness, targeting revision to
    8–9
assessment
    of capacity 33, 45–6
    and OSCE 33, 45–6
    and patient management problems 140–2
ataxia 12
atenolol 21
atropine 21
autistic spectrum disorder 140–2
Autonomy vs Shame and Doubt stage 17

barbiturates 15
Bateson, G. 15
Baumeister, R. 15
Beck, A. 15
belongingness 15
benzisoxazoles 22
bias in research studies 48, 64
bilateral temporal lobe 18
bipolar affective disorder 79
    sample essay 114–17
blood tests 144–5
books
    on critical review 50, 55
    of ISQ/EMI questions and answers 9
    medical textbooks 34
    and OSCE 34
    for Part I 2
    for Part II 2
    patient management problems
        practice books 144
    on psychiatric examination 34, 157

caffeine consumption, and exams 4
CAGE questionnaire 32, 33
calculated measures, in critical review 49,
    53–4, 56–9
calculators 49
capacity assessments, in OSCE 33, 45–6
carers 87–8, 118–22
case conferences 142
case–control studies 63–4
'Changing Minds' campaign 86–7
child psychiatry 132–7, 140–2
chlorpromazine 22
cognitive function, assessment in OSCE 33
cognitive triad 15
cohort studies 62–3
communication skills, and OSCE 44
community care 111–13
conditioned response 24
conditioning 24
confabulation 18
consent, capacity assessment in OSCE 33, 45
control event rate (CER) 58
control groups 61
critical discussion of information 68–9
critical review 47–64
    approach to paper 51–2
    bibliography 55
    defined 47
    and formulae 56–9
    marking 51–2
    past papers 50
    preparation 48–50
        knowledge 48–50
        practice 50
        skills 50
    Question A 52–4
    Question B 54
    Royal College view 47–8
    and study designs 60–4
    time available 51
curriculum 7–8
cyclopyrrolones 22

'Defeat Depression' campaign 86
defence mechanisms 15
delirium tremens 12
dementia 13, 118–22

84–5
negative predictive value (NPV) 49, 57
neocortex 15
number needed to treat (NNT) 49, 53,
    59

object relations theorists 12
obsessive–compulsive disorder 80
occipital lobe 18
odds ratio (OR) 49, 59
old age psychiatry
    National Service Framework for Older
        People 84–5
    sample essays 118–27
oral stage 19
organic causes 145, 146, 156
OSCE (Objective Structured Clinical
    Examination) 27–46
    advantages/disadvantages 27–8
    assessments of capacity 33, 45–6
    common mistakes/pitfalls 45
    common scenarios 42–4
    exam day 34–41
        booths 35–6
        conduct of station 37–41
        cycles of stations 35
        dealing with actors 36–7
        examiners 35, 36, 38
        finishing the station 41
        introductions 38–9
        negotiating the exam 41
        pilot stations 36
        reading the question 38
        rest stations 36
        setting the scene 39
        speaking 37–8
        tackling the question 40
        venues 35
    marking scheme 28–9, 37
    practice of scenarios 34
    preparation and revision technique
        29–34
        factual knowledge 29–32
        physical examination and practical
            skills 33–4
        psychiatric clinical skills 32–3
        use of structural frameworks 29–30,
            31, 32
    Royal College view 28–9
    skills tested 28, 33
    stations 27, 28, 35, 36, 37–41
outcome measures 62

panic disorder 79
Part I
    and curriculum 8
    extended matching items (EMIs) 7–25
    individual statement questions (ISQs)
        7–25
        sample ISQs 12–13
    OSCE 27–46
    useful books 2
Part II
    clinical 139, 149
    critical review 47–64
    essay 65–137
    extended matching items (EMIs) 7–25
    individual statement questions (ISQs)
        7–25
        basic sciences sample ISQs 15
        clinical topics sample ISQs 14
    long case 149–63
    patient management problems 139–47
    useful books 2
'Partners in Care' campaign 87–8
patient management problems (PMPs)
    139–47
    arguing with examiners 147
    and case conferences 142
    and collateral information 146
    and emergency situations 143, 146
    example 140–2
    exam techniques 144–7
    group working 4, 140
    and investigations 144–5
    and multidisciplinary working 140–1
    and patient assessment 140–2
    practice books and sessions 140, 144
    probes 146–7
    revision techniques 139–44
pencil marks 11
pens 66
perception 15
perseveration 12
personality disorder 80–1
    sample essay 106–10
personality theories, idiographic 25
phenothiazines, aliphatic 22
physical examination
    and long case 157, 158
    and OSCE 33–4
Piaget, J. 19
planning revision 1–5
positive predictive value (PPV) 49, 53, 56–7
post-traumatic stress disorder 80